FACTS
OF LIFE AND
DEATH

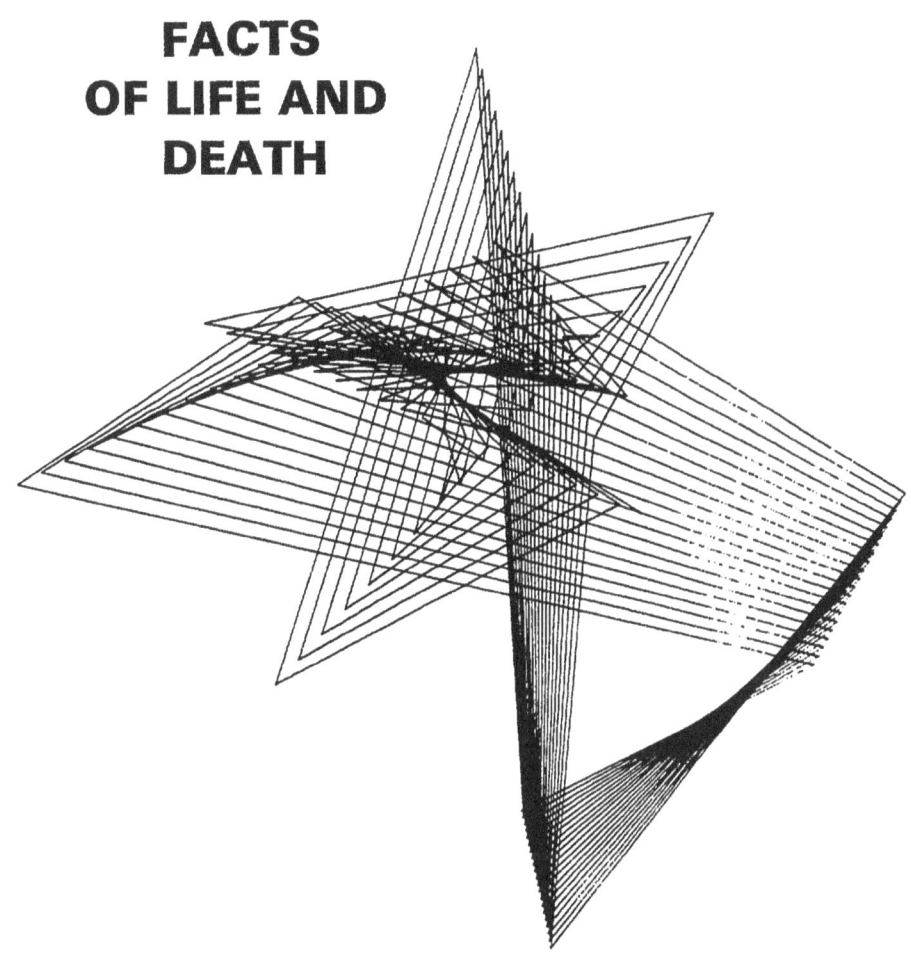

DHEW Publication No. (PHS) 79-1222

U.S. DEPARTMENT OF HEALTH, EDUCATION, AND WELFARE
Public Health Service
National Center for Health Statistics
Hyattsville, Maryland 20782
November 1978

NATIONAL CENTER FOR HEALTH STATISTICS

DOROTHY P. RICE, *Director*

ROBERT A. ISRAEL, *Deputy Director*
JACOB J. FELDMAN, Ph.D., *Associate Director for Analysis*
GAIL F. FISHER, Ph.D., *Associate Director for the Cooperative Health Statistics Systems*
ELIJAH L. WHITE, *Associate Director for Data Systems*
JAMES T. BAIRD, JR., Ph.D., *Associate Director for International Statistics*
ROBERT C. HUBER, *Associate Director for Management*
MONROE G. SIRKEN, Ph.D., *Associate Director for Mathematical Statistics*
PETER L. HURLEY, *Associate Director for Operations*
JAMES M. ROBEY, Ph.D., *Associate Director for Program Development*
PAUL E. LEAVERTON, Ph.D., *Associate Director for Research*
ALICE HAYWOOD, *Information Officer*

DHEW Publication No. (PHS) 79-1222

Library of Congress Catalog Card Number 74-4020

CONTENTS

Introduction   1

I. Population

Table 1. Population residing in the United States and annual rate of increase (percent per year) between dates given: Selected years, 1900-1976   2

Table 2. Population residing in the United States, by age, and percent distribution of total population in each age group: 1940, 1960, 1970, and 1976   2

II. Births

Chart A. Birth rates: 1930-76   3

Table 3. Live births and birth rates: Selected years, 1930-76   3

Chart B. Fertility rates: 1930-76   4

Table 4. Birth rates by age of mother: Selected years, 1940-76   4

Chart C. Estimated illegitimacy rates: 1940-76   5

Table 5. Estimated number of illegitimate live births and illegitimacy rates and ratios: Selected years, 1940-76   5

III. Life Expectancy

Table 6. Average remaining lifetime in years at specified ages: Selected years, 1900-1902 to 1976 . . .   6

Table 7. Average remaining lifetime in years at specified ages, by color and sex: 1900-1902, 1969-71, and 1976   7

IV. Fetal, Infant, and Maternal Mortality

Table 8. Fetal deaths and fetal death ratios: Selected years, 1945-76   8

Table 9. Infant and maternal mortality: Selected years, 1935-76   8

Chart D. Infant mortality rates: 1930-76   9

Table 10. Neonatal mortality rates by color and sex: Selected years, 1950-76   9

V. Marriage and Divorce

Chart E. Marriage and divorce rates: 1930-76   10

Table 11. Marriages, divorces, and rates: Selected years, 1930-76   10

VI. Health Characteristics

Table 12. Selected health statistics: 1975   11

Table 13. Leading causes of bed disability due to acute conditions: 1975   12

Table 14. Number of persons with limitation of activity by selected chronic conditions causing limitation: 1974   13

Table 15. Communicable diseases—reported cases and registered deaths: 1969-76   14

Table 16. Dental, sensory, and speech defects in youths aged 12-17 years: 1966-70   16

Table 17. Dental, sensory, and speech defects in children age 6-11 years: 1963-65   17

Table 18. Prevalence rates of heart disease, hypertension, and arthritis in adults by age and sex: 1960-62   18

VII. Physical Measurements

Table 19. Weight range of men and women by age and height: 1960-62 19
Table 20. Weight range of boys and girls 6-17 years of age by single year of age and height: 1963-70... 20

VIII. Health Resources

Table 21. Estimated persons employed in selected occupations within each health field: 1974 22
Table 22. Physicians in relation to population: Selected years, 1950-76......................... 26
Table 23. Physicians by type of practice: Selected years, 1968-74 28

IX. Mortality

General

Chart F. Death rates: 1930-76 29
Table 24. Deaths, death rates, and age-adjusted death rates: Selected years, 1935-76 29
Table 25. Deaths and death rates by age and sex: 1976 30

Leading Causes

Table 26. Deaths and death rates for the 10 leading causes of death in 1976 and death rates for these same causes in 1900 31
Table 27. Deaths and death rates for the 10 leading causes of death, by sex: 1976 32
Table 28. Deaths and death rates for the 10 leading causes of death in specified age and sex groups: 1976 33

Selected Causes

Table 29. Age-adjusted death rates for 69 selected causes of death: 1970 and 1976 39
Table 30. Death rates for Diseases of heart by color and sex: Selected years, 1950-76 41
Table 31. Deaths and death rates for Diseases of heart by age and sex: 1976 41
Table 32. Death rates for Malignant neoplasms, including neoplasms of lymphatic and hematopoietic tissues by color and sex: Selected years, 1950-76.................................... 42
Table 33. Deaths and death rates for Malignant neoplasms, including neoplasms of lymphatic and hematopoietic tissues by age and sex: 1976 42
Table 34. Death rates for Cerebrovascular diseases by color and sex: Selected years, 1950-76 43
Table 35. Death rates for Arteriosclerosis by color and sex: Selected years, 1950-76............... 43
Table 36. Death rates for Bronchitis, emphysema, and asthma by color and sex: Selected years, 1950-76 44
Table 37. Deaths and death rates for Bronchitis, emphysema, and asthma by age and sex: 1976 44
Table 38. Death rates for Accidents by color and sex: Selected years, 1950-76 45
Table 39. Deaths and death rates for Motor vehicle accidents and All other accidents in order of frequency: 1976 45
Table 40. Death rates for Suicide by color and sex: Selected years, 1950-76 46
Table 41. Deaths and death rates for Suicide by age and sex: 1976 46
Table 42. Death rates for Homicide by color and sex: Selected years, 1950-76 47
Table 43. Death rates for Homicide by age and sex: 1976 47

SYMBOLS

Data not available--	- - -
Category not applicable------------------------------------	. . .
Quantity zero--	-
Quantity more than 0 but less than 0.05------	0.0
Figure does not meet standards of reliability or precision---------------------------	*

INTRODUCTION

The statistics in this report have been assembled by the National Center for Health Statistics to answer questions frequently asked about vital and health statistics for the United States.

Information on births, deaths, marriages, divorces, and life expectancy is based on vital data gathered by the Center's Division of Vital Statistics from the individual States, which are responsible for the registration of these events.

With one exception, the data on health characteristics of the U.S. population are based upon surveys conducted by the Center's Division of Health Interview Statistics and Division of Health Examination Statistics. The exception is reported cases of communicable diseases, which are compiled by the Center for Disease Control, Public Health Service, Atlanta, Georgia.

Data on health personnel are gathered by the Center's Division of Health Resources Utilization Statistics primarily from professional associations.

Vital statistics shown in this report include only events occurring within a specified area. Beginning with 1933, all data cover events occurring within the entire conterminous (48) United States. Beginning with 1959, the figures include Alaska, and starting with 1960, they include Hawaii. For the years prior to 1933, data for marriages, divorces, and births, when these are shown as having been adjusted for underregistration, are for the entire United States. Data for registered births and deaths prior to 1933 are for expanding groups of registration States. Beginning with 1970, data exclude births and deaths of nonresidents of the United States. In that year there were 6,414 births to nonresidents and 1,935 deaths of nonresidents.

Fetal deaths are excluded from birth and death statistics. Fetal death figures for 1969-76 include only fetal deaths for which the stated or presumed period of gestation was 20 weeks or more. For earlier years gestational age not stated is included.

Numbers shown as estimated in certain vital statistics tables are based on a sample of incomplete data. Numbers shown as provisional are based on figures reported on a monthly basis and are subject to revision in final tabulations.

Rates are based on population figures from the U.S. Bureau of the Census. Birth and divorce rates for 1941-46 are based on population including the Armed Forces abroad; other rates are based on total population residing in the area. Beginning with 1940 for years ending in a zero, rates are based on the enumerated population as indicated in table 1. For all other years, rates are based on estimated midyear population.

I. POPULATION

Table 1. Population residing in the United States and annual rate of increase (percent per year) between dates given: Selected years, 1900-1976

Year	Population	Annual rate of increase
1976 (estimated as of July 1)---	214,649,000	0.76
1975 (estimated as of July 1)---	213,032,000	0.78
1974 (estimated as of July 1)---	211,390,000	0.73
1973 (estimated as of July 1)---	209,851,000	0.78
1972 (estimated as of July 1)---	208,230,000	0.98
1971 (estimated as of July 1)---	206,212,000	1.18
1970 (19th decennial census, April 1)--------------------------------	203,211,926	1.21
1969 (estimated as of July 1)---	201,385,000	1.00
1968 (estimated as of July 1)---	199,399,000	0.98
1967 (estimated as of July 1)---	197,457,000	0.96
1966 (estimated as of July 1)---	195,576,000	1.06
1965 (estimated as of July 1)---	193,526,000	1.46
1960 (18th decennial census, April 1)--------------------------------	179,323,175	1.75
1950 (17th decennial census, April 1)--------------------------------	150,697,361	1.36
1940 (16th decennial census, April 1)--------------------------------	131,669,275	0.70
1930 (15th decennial census, April 1)--------------------------------	122,775,046	1.47
1920 (14th decennial census, Jan. 1)---------------------------------	105,710,620	1.44
1910 (13th decennial census, April 15)-------------------------------	91,972,266	1.95
1900 (12th decennial census, June 1)---------------------------------	75,994,575	...

Table 2. Population residing in the United States, by age, and percent distribution of total population in each age group: 1940, 1960, 1970, and 1976

[Enumerated as of April 1 for 1940, 1960, and 1970 and estimated as of July 1 for 1976]

Age	Population in millions				Percent of total population in age group			
	1976	1970	1960	1940	1976	1970	1960	1940
All ages------------------------------	214.6	203.2	179.3	131.7	100.0	100.0	100.0	100.0
Under 5 years--------------------------------	15.3	17.2	20.3	10.5	7.1	8.4	11.3	8.0
5-9 years----------------------------------	17.3	20.0	18.7	10.7	8.1	9.8	10.4	8.1
10-14 years--------------------------------	19.8	20.8	16.8	11.7	9.2	10.2	9.4	8.9
15-19 years--------------------------------	21.2	19.1	13.2	12.3	9.9	9.4	7.4	9.4
20-24 years--------------------------------	19.4	16.4	10.8	11.6	9.1	8.1	6.0	8.8
25-29 years--------------------------------	17.7	13.5	10.9	11.1	8.3	6.6	6.1	8.4
30-34 years--------------------------------	14.2	11.4	11.9	10.2	6.6	5.6	6.7	7.8
35-39 years--------------------------------	11.9	11.1	12.5	9.5	5.5	5.5	7.0	7.2
40-44 years--------------------------------	11.1	12.0	11.6	8.8	5.2	5.9	6.5	6.7
45-49 years--------------------------------	11.7	12.1	10.9	8.3	5.4	6.0	6.1	6.3
50-54 years--------------------------------	12.0	11.1	9.6	7.3	5.6	5.5	5.4	5.5
55-59 years--------------------------------	10.8	10.0	8.4	5.9	5.0	4.9	4.7	4.5
60-64 years--------------------------------	9.3	8.6	7.1	4.8	4.3	4.2	4.0	3.6
65-69 years--------------------------------	8.3	7.0	6.3	3.8	3.9	3.4	3.5	2.9
70-74 years--------------------------------	5.9	5.4	4.7	2.6	2.8	2.7	2.6	2.0
75 years and over--------------------------	8.7	7.6	5.6	2.6	4.1	3.8	3.1	2.0

II. BIRTHS

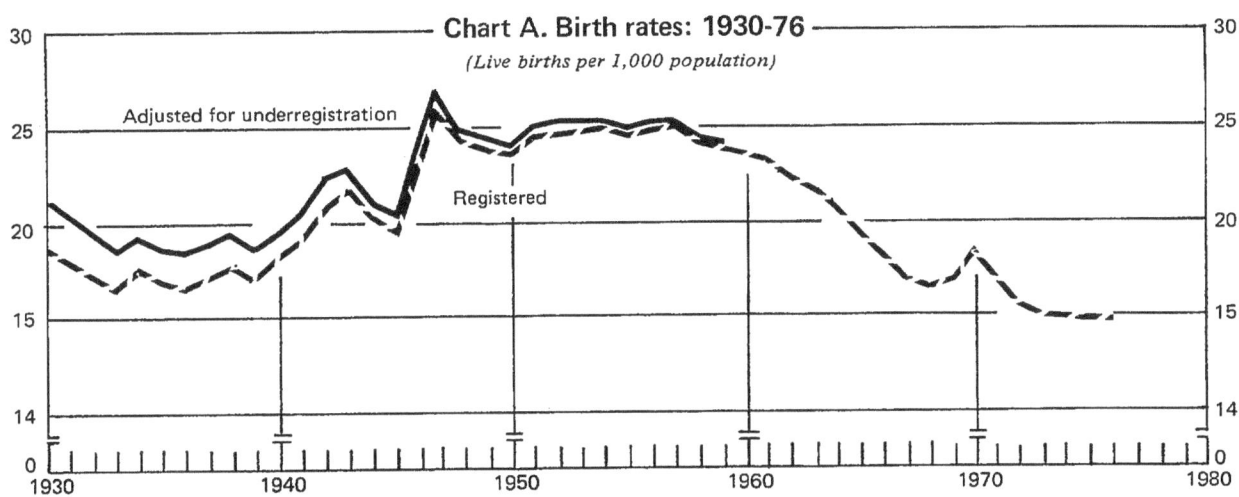

Chart A. Birth rates: 1930-76
(Live births per 1,000 population)

Adjusted for underregistration

Registered

Table 3. Live births and birth rates: Selected years, 1930-76

Year	Registered live births[1]		Births adjusted for underregistration[2]	
	Number	Rate per 1,000 population	Number	Rate per 1,000 population
1976[3]	3,167,788	14.8	---	---
1975[3]	3,144,198	14.8	---	---
1974[3]	3,159,958	14.9	---	---
1973[3]	3,136,965	14.9	---	---
1972[3]	3,258,411	15.6	---	---
1971[4]	3,555,970	17.2	---	---
1970[4]	3,731,386	18.4	---	---
1969[4]	3,600,206	[a]17.9	---	---
1968[4]	3,501,564	[a]17.6	---	---
1967[5]	3,520,959	17.8	---	---
1966[4]	3,606,274	18.4	---	---
1965[4]	3,760,358	19.4	---	---
1960[4]	4,257,850	23.7	---	---
1955	4,047,295	24.6	4,097,000	25.0
1950	3,554,149	23.6	3,632,000	24.1
1945	2,735,456	19.5	2,858,000	20.4
1940	2,360,399	17.9	2,559,000	19.4
1935	2,155,105	16.9	2,377,000	18.7
1930	[6]2,203,958	18.9	[7]2,618,000	21.3

[1]Beginning in 1970, excludes births to nonresidents of the United States.
[2]Adjustment for underregistration discontinued after 1959.
[3]Based on 100 percent of births in selected States and on a 50-percent sample of births in all other States.
[4]Based on a 50-percent sample of births.
[5]Based on a 20- to 50-percent sample of births.
[6]Birth-registration area included 46 States.
[7]Estimated for the entire United States.
[a]Revised.

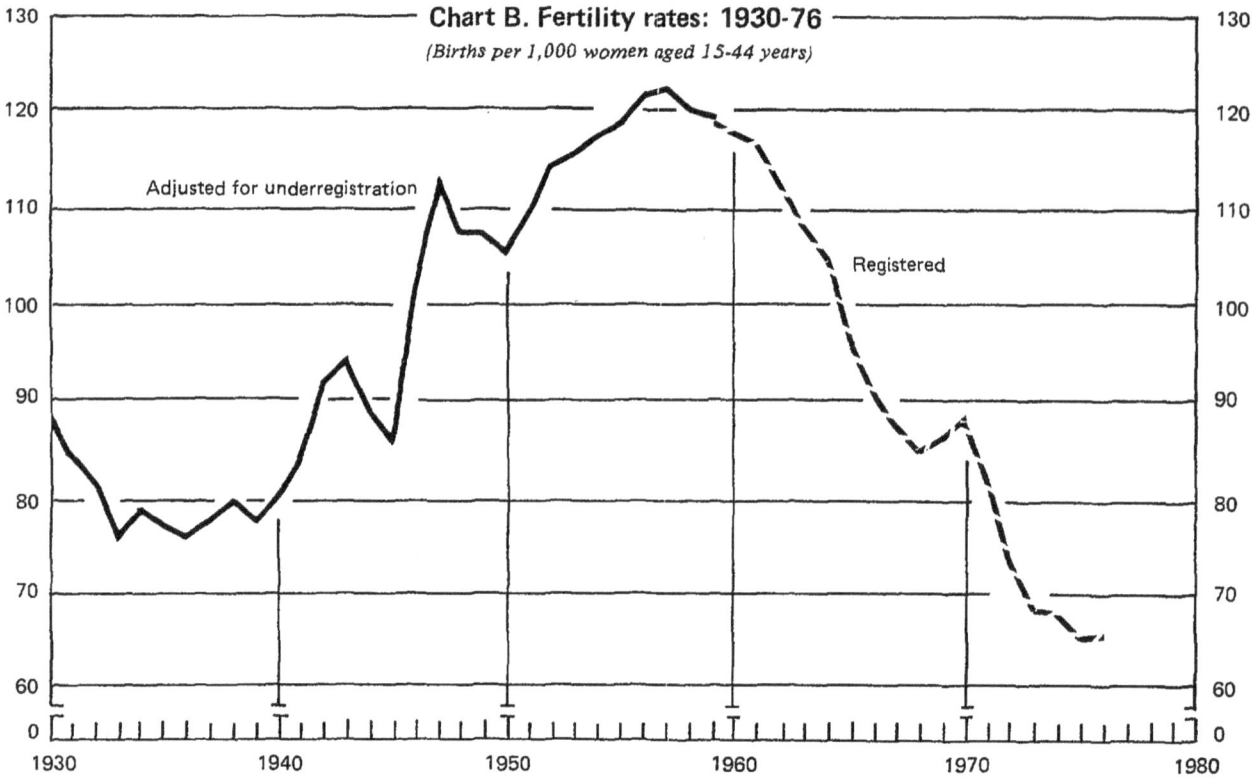

Chart B. Fertility rates: 1930-76

(Births per 1,000 women aged 15-44 years)

Adjusted for underregistration

Registered

Table 4. Birth rates by age of mother: Selected years, 1940-76

[Rates per 1,000 female population in specified groups]

Year	15-44 years[1]	10-14 years	15-19 years	20-24 years	25-29 years	30-34 years	35-39 years	40-44 years	45-49 years
1976 [2,3]	65.8	1.2	53.5	112.1	108.8	54.5	19.0	4.3	0.2
1975 [2,3]	66.7	1.3	56.3	114.7	110.3	53.1	19.4	4.6	0.3
1974 [2,3]	68.4	1.2	58.1	119.0	113.3	54.4	20.2	4.8	0.3
1973 [2,3]	69.2	1.3	59.7	120.7	113.6	56.1	22.0	5.4	0.3
1972 [2,3]	73.4	1.2	62.0	131.0	118.7	60.2	24.8	6.2	0.4
1971 [2,4]	81.8	1.1	64.7	150.6	134.8	67.6	28.7	7.1	0.4
1970 [2,4]	87.9	1.2	68.3	167.8	145.1	73.3	31.7	8.1	0.5
1969 [4,a]	86.1	1.0	65.5	165.7	143.0	73.5	33.1	8.8	0.5
1968 [4,a]	85.2	1.0	65.6	166.5	140.0	74.2	35.4	9.6	0.6
1967 [5,a]	87.2	0.9	67.5	172.9	142.1	78.7	38.3	10.6	0.7
1966 [4,a]	90.8	0.8	70.3	185.6	148.2	85.1	41.9	11.7	0.7
1965 [4,a]	96.3	0.8	70.5	195.3	161.6	94.4	46.2	12.8	0.8
1960 [4]	118.0	0.8	89.1	258.1	197.4	112.7	56.2	15.5	0.9
1955	118.3	0.9	90.3	241.6	190.2	116.0	58.6	16.1	1.0
1950	106.2	1.0	81.6	196.6	166.1	103.7	52.9	15.1	1.2
1945	85.9	0.8	51.1	138.9	132.2	100.2	56.9	16.6	1.6
1940	79.9	0.7	54.1	135.6	122.8	83.4	46.3	15.6	1.9

[1] Computed relating total births, regardless of age of mother, to women aged 15-44 years.
[2] Excludes births to nonresidents of the United States.
[3] Based on 100 percent of births in selected States and on a 50-percent sample of births in all other States.
[4] Based on a 50-percent sample of births.
[5] Based on a 20- to 50-percent sample of births.
[a] Revised.

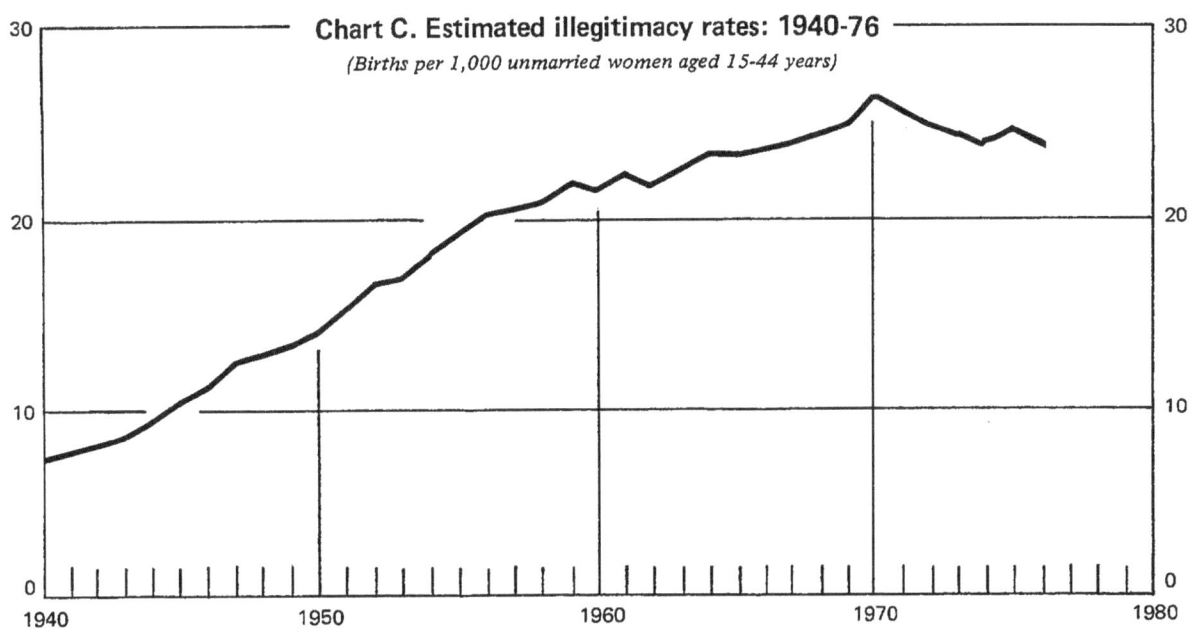

Chart C. Estimated illegitimacy rates: 1940-76
(Births per 1,000 unmarried women aged 15-44 years)

Table 5. Estimated number of illegitimate live births and illegitimacy rates and ratios: Selected years, 1940-76

Year	Number	Rate per 1,000 unmarried women aged 15-44 years	Ratio per 1,000 total live births
1976 [1,2]	468,100	24.7	147.8
1975 [1,2]	447,900	24.8	142.5
1974 [1,2]	418,100	24.1	132.3
1973 [1,2]	407,300	24.5	129.8
1972 [1,2]	403,200	24.9	123.7
1971 [1,3]	401,400	25.6	112.9
1970 [1,3]	398,700	[a]26.4	106.9
1969 [3]	360,800	[a]24.8	100.2
1968 [3]	339,200	[a]24.3	96.9
1967 [4]	318,100	[a]23.7	90.3
1966 [3]	302,400	[a]23.3	83.9
1965 [3]	291,200	[a]23.4	77.4
1960 [3]	224,300	21.6	52.7
1955	183,300	19.3	45.3
1950	141,600	14.1	39.8
1945	117,400	10.1	42.9
1940	89,500	7.1	37.9

[1]Excludes births to nonresidents of the United States.
[2]Based on 100 percent of births in selected States and on a 50-percent sample of births in all other States.
[3]Based on a 50-percent sample of births.
[4]Based on a 20- to 50-percent sample of births.
[a]Revised.

5

III. LIFE EXPECTANCY

Table 6. Average remaining lifetime in years at specified ages: Selected years, 1900-1902 to 1976

[For 1900-1902, data are for 10 States and the District of Columbia; for 1919-21, for 34 States and the District of Columbia. Beginning with 1939-41, data are for the United States]

Age in years	1976	1969-71	1959-61	1949-51	1939-41	1919-21	1900-1902
0-----------------------------------	72.8	70.75	69.89	68.07	63.62	56.40	49.24
1-----------------------------------	72.9	71.19	70.75	69.16	65.76	59.94	55.20
5-----------------------------------	69.1	67.43	67.04	65.54	62.49	57.99	54.98
10----------------------------------	64.2	62.57	62.19	60.74	57.82	53.79	51.14
15----------------------------------	59.3	57.69	57.33	55.91	53.10	49.37	46.81
20----------------------------------	54.6	53.00	52.58	51.20	48.54	45.30	42.79
25----------------------------------	50.0	48.37	47.89	46.56	44.09	41.47	39.12
30----------------------------------	45.3	43.71	43.18	41.91	39.67	37.68	35.51
35----------------------------------	40.6	39.07	38.51	37.31	35.30	33.89	31.92
40----------------------------------	35.9	34.52	33.92	32.81	31.03	30.08	28.34
45----------------------------------	31.5	30.12	29.50	28.49	26.90	26.25	24.77
50----------------------------------	27.2	25.93	25.29	24.40	22.98	22.50	21.26
55----------------------------------	23.2	21.99	21.37	20.57	19.31	18.90	17.88
60----------------------------------	19.4	18.34	17.71	17.04	15.91	15.54	14.76
65----------------------------------	16.0	15.00	14.39	13.83	12.80	12.47	11.86
70----------------------------------	12.9	12.00	11.38	10.92	10.00	9.74	9.30
75----------------------------------	10.1	9.32	8.71	8.40	7.62	7.49	7.08
80----------------------------------	7.9	7.10	6.39	6.34	5.73	---	5.30
85----------------------------------	6.1	5.28	4.58	4.69	4.31	---	3.96

Table 7. Average remaining lifetime in years at specified ages, by color and sex: 1900-1902, 1969-71, and 1976

[For 1900-1902, data are for 10 States and the District of Columbia; for 1969-71 and 1976 data are for the United States]

Age in years	1976	1969-71	1900-1902[1]	1976	1969-71	1900-1902[1]
	White, male			White, female		
0---	69.7	67.94	48.23	77.3	75.49	51.08
1---	69.8	68.33	54.61	77.2	75.66	56.39
5---	66.0	64.55	54.43	73.4	71.86	56.03
10--	61.1	59.69	50.59	68.5	66.97	52.15
15--	56.2	54.83	46.25	63.6	62.07	47.79
20--	51.6	50.22	42.19	58.7	57.24	43.77
25--	47.1	45.70	38.52	53.9	52.42	40.05
30--	42.4	41.07	34.88	49.1	47.60	36.42
35--	37.7	36.43	31.29	44.2	42.82	32.82
40--	33.1	31.87	27.74	39.5	38.12	29.17
45--	28.7	27.48	24.21	34.9	33.54	25.51
50--	24.4	23.34	20.76	30.4	29.11	21.89
55--	20.5	19.51	17.42	26.1	24.85	18.43
60--	16.9	16.07	14.35	22.0	20.79	15.23
65--	13.7	13.02	11.51	18.1	16.93	12.23
70--	10.9	10.38	9.03	14.4	13.37	9.59
75--	8.5	8.06	6.84	11.2	10.21	7.33
80--	6.6	6.18	5.10	8.5	7.59	5.50
85--	5.1	4.63	3.81	6.4	5.54	4.10
	All other, male			All other, female		
0---	64.1	60.98	32.54	72.6	69.05	35.04
1---	64.9	62.13	42.46	73.3	70.01	43.54
5---	61.1	58.48	45.06	69.5	66.34	46.04
10--	56.3	53.67	41.90	64.6	61.49	43.02
15--	51.4	48.84	38.26	59.7	56.60	39.79
20--	46.8	44.37	35.11	54.9	51.85	36.89
25--	42.5	40.29	32.21	50.2	47.19	33.90
30--	38.2	36.20	29.25	45.5	42.61	30.70
35--	34.0	32.16	26.16	40.9	38.14	27.52
40--	30.0	28.29	23.12	36.4	33.87	24.37
45--	26.1	24.64	20.09	32.1	29.80	21.36
50--	22.5	21.24	17.34	28.0	25.97	18.67
55--	19.2	18.14	14.69	24.3	22.37	15.88
60--	16.3	15.35	12.62	20.7	19.02	13.60
65--	13.8	12.87	10.38	17.6	15.99	11.38
70--	11.3	10.68	8.33	14.3	13.30	9.62
75--	9.7	8.99	6.60	12.3	11.06	7.90
80--	8.6	7.57	5.12	10.9	9.01	6.48
85--	7.2	6.04	4.04	9.1	7.07	5.10

[1] Figures for the All other group cover only Negroes. However, the Negro population comprised 95 percent of the corresponding All other population.

IV. FETAL, INFANT, AND MATERNAL MORTALITY

There is substantial evidence that many fetal deaths are not reported. Consequently, the ratios shown in table 8 are believed to be considerably understated. These are annual national estimates based on the registered births and fetal deaths. Birth registration is much more complete than fetal death registration.

Table 8. Fetal deaths and fetal death ratios: Selected years, 1945-76

[Fetal deaths for 1969-76 include only those with stated or presumed gestation of 20 weeks or more. For earlier years gestational age not stated is included]

Year	Number	Ratio per 1,000 live births	Year	Number	Ratio per 1,000 live births
1976	33,111	10.5	1968	55,293	15.8
1975	33,796	10.7	1967	54,934	15.6
1974	36,281	11.5	1966	56,637	15.7
1973	38,309	12.2	1965	60,859	16.2
1972	41,380	12.7	1960	68,480	16.1
1971	47,818	13.4	1955	69,153	17.1
1970	52,961	14.2	1950	68,262	19.2
1969	50,749	14.1	1945	65,513	23.9

Table 9. Infant and maternal mortality: Selected years, 1935-76

Year	Infant mortality				Maternal mortality[1]			
	Number of deaths under 1 year	Rate per 1,000 live births			Number of maternal deaths	Rate per 100,000 live births		
		Total	White	All other		Total	White	All other
1976[2]	48,265	15.2	13.3	23.5	390	12.3	9.0	26.5
1975[2]	50,525	16.1	14.2	24.2	403	12.8	9.1	29.0
1974[2]	52,776	16.7	14.8	24.9	462	14.6	10.0	35.1
1973[2]	55,581	17.7	15.8	26.2	477	15.2	10.7	34.6
1972[2,3]	60,182	18.5	16.4	27.7	612	18.8	14.3	38.5
1971[2]	67,981	19.1	17.1	28.5	668	18.8	13.0	45.3
1970[2]	74,667	20.0	17.8	30.9	803	21.5	14.4	55.9
1969	75,073	20.9	18.4	32.9	801	22.2	15.5	55.7
1968	76,263	21.8	19.2	34.5	859	24.5	16.6	63.6
1967	79,028	22.4	19.7	35.9	987	28.0	19.5	69.5
1966	85,516	23.7	20.6	38.8	1,049	29.1	20.2	72.4
1965	92,866	24.7	21.5	40.3	1,189	31.6	21.0	83.7
1960	110,873	26.0	22.9	43.2	1,579	37.1	26.0	97.9
1955	106,903	26.4	23.6	42.8	1,901	47.0	32.8	130.3
1950	103,825	29.2	26.8	44.5	2,960	83.3	61.1	221.6
1945	104,684	38.3	35.6	57.0	5,668	207.2	172.1	454.8
1940	110,984	47.0	43.2	73.8	8,876	376.0	319.8	773.5
1935	120,138	55.7	51.9	83.7	12,544	582.1	530.6	945.7

[1] Refers to deaths from Complications of pregnancy, childbirth, and the puerperium.
[2] Excludes deaths of nonresidents of the United States.
[3] Based on a 50-percent sample of deaths.

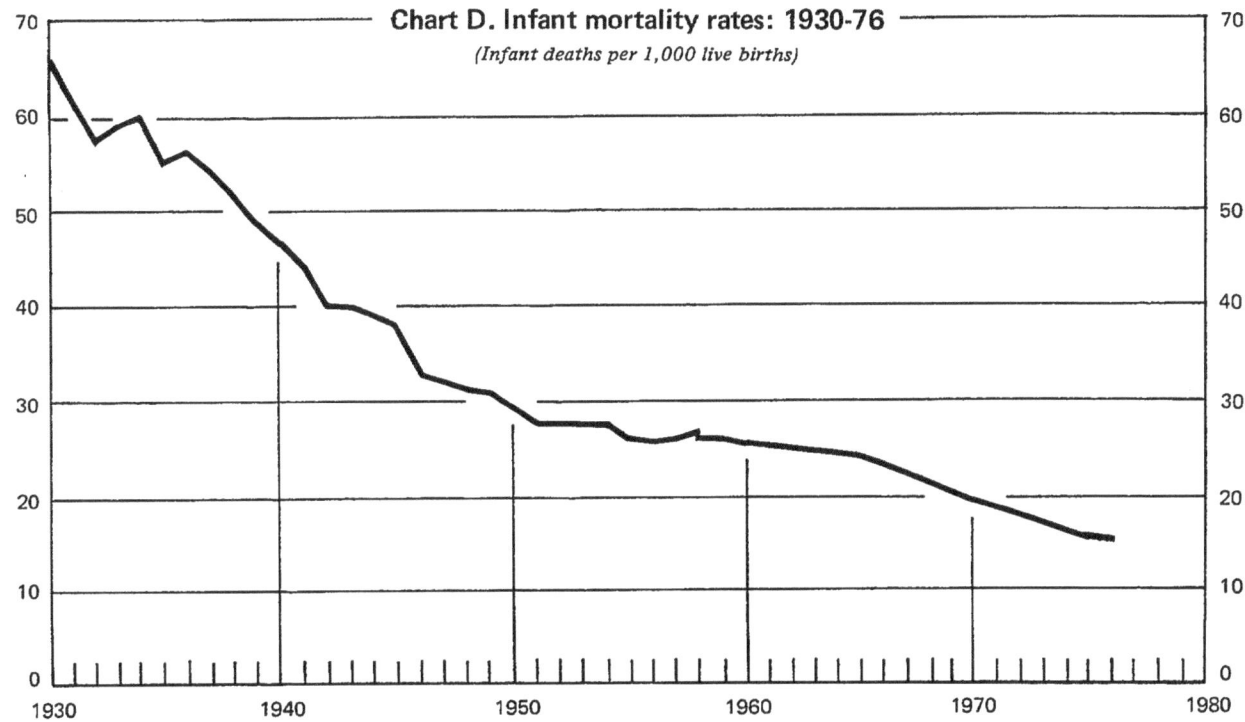

Chart D. Infant mortality rates: 1930-76
(Infant deaths per 1,000 live births)

Table 10. Neonatal mortality rates by color and sex: Selected years, 1950-76
[Rates are deaths under 28 days per 1,000 live births in specified color-sex group]

Year	Number of deaths under 28 days	Total			White			All other		
		Both sexes	Male	Female	Both sexes	Male	Female	Both sexes	Male	Female
1976[1] --------------	34,587	10.9	12.0	9.7	9.7	10.7	8.5	16.3	17.7	14.9
1975[1] --------------	36,416	11.6	12.9	10.2	10.4	11.7	9.0	16.8	18.2	15.3
1974[1] --------------	38,738	12.3	13.8	10.7	11.1	12.6	9.6	17.2	18.9	15.4
1973[1] --------------	40,664	13.0	14.6	11.2	11.8	13.5	10.1	17.9	19.8	15.9
1972[1,2] ------------	44,432	13.6	15.4	11.7	12.4	14.1	10.5	19.2	21.2	17.2
1971[1] --------------	50,496	14.2	16.0	12.3	13.0	14.8	11.2	19.6	21.9	17.2
1970[1] --------------	56,279	15.1	17.0	13.1	13.8	15.5	11.9	21.4	23.9	18.9
1969--------------	56,085	15.6	17.7	13.3	14.2	16.2	12.0	22.5	25.3	19.8
1968--------------	56,456	16.1	18.3	13.8	14.7	16.9	12.4	23.0	25.5	20.4
1967--------------	58,127	16.5	18.7	14.2	15.0	17.2	12.7	23.8	26.3	21.2
1966--------------	61,941	17.2	19.5	14.8	15.6	17.9	13.2	24.8	27.5	22.1
1965--------------	66,419	17.7	20.0	15.2	16.1	18.3	13.8	25.4	28.4	22.4
1960--------------	79,733	18.7	21.2	16.1	17.2	19.7	14.7	26.9	30.0	23.6
1955--------------	77,351	19.1	21.7	16.4	17.7	20.3	15.1	27.2	30.2	24.1
1950--------------	72,855	20.5	23.3	17.5	19.4	22.2	16.4	27.5	30.8	24.2

[1]Excludes deaths of nonresidents of the United States.
[2]Based on a 50-percent sample of deaths.

V. MARRIAGE AND DIVORCE

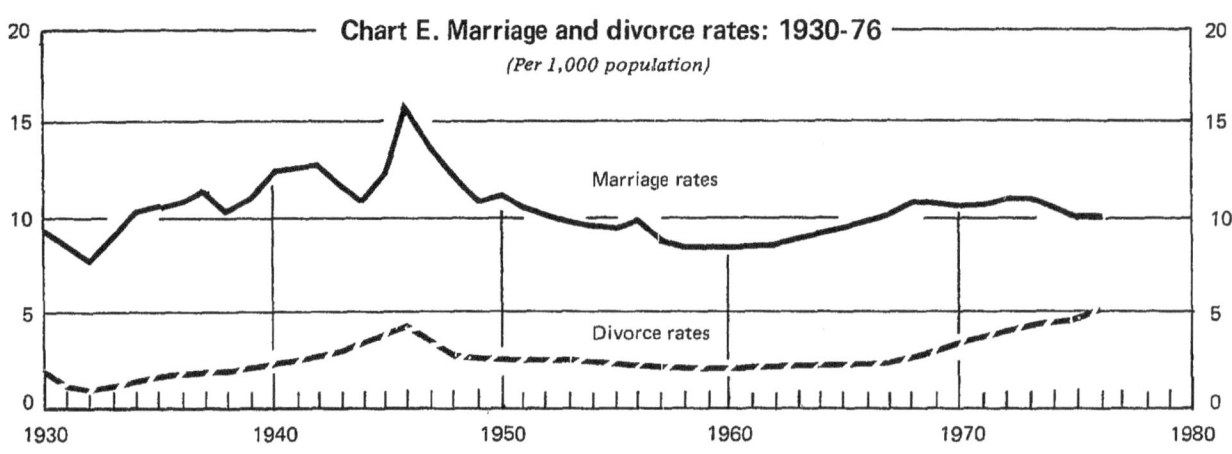

Chart E. Marriage and divorce rates: 1930-76
(Per 1,000 population)

Table 11. Marriages, divorces, and rates: Selected years, 1930-76

Year	Marriages[1]				Divorces[2]		
	Number	Rate per 1,000 population	Rate per 1,000 unmarried women 15-44 years	Rate per 1,000 unmarried women 15 years and over	Number	Rate per 1,000 population	Rate per 1,000 married women 15 years and over
1976------------------------	2,154,807	10.0	113.4	65.2	1,083,000	5.0	21.1
1975------------------------	2,152,662	10.1	118.5	66.9	1,036,000	4.9	20.3
1974------------------------	2,229,667	10.5	128.4	72.0	977,000	4.6	19.3
1973------------------------	2,284,108	10.9	137.3	76.0	915,000	4.4	18.2
1972------------------------	2,282,154	11.0	141.3	77.9	845,000	4.1	17.0
1971------------------------	2,190,481	10.6	138.9	76.2	773,000	3.7	15.8
1970------------------------	2,158,802	10.6	140.2	76.5	708,000	3.5	14.9
1969------------------------	2,145,000	10.6	149.1	80.0	639,000	3.2	13.4
1968------------------------	2,069,000	10.4	147.2	79.1	584,000	2.9	12.5
1967------------------------	1,927,000	9.7	145.2	76.4	523,000	2.6	11.2
1966------------------------	1,857,000	9.5	145.1	75.6	499,000	2.5	10.9
1965------------------------	1,800,000	9.3	144.3	75.0	479,000	2.5	10.6
1960------------------------	1,523,000	8.5	148.0	73.5	393,000	2.2	9.2
1955------------------------	1,531,000	9.3	161.1	80.9	377,000	2.3	9.3
1950------------------------	1,667,231	11.1	166.4	90.2	385,144	2.6	10.3
1945------------------------	1,612,992	12.2	138.2	83.6	485,000	3.5	14.4
1940------------------------	1,595,879	12.1	127.4	82.8	264,000	2.0	8.8
1935------------------------	1,327,000	10.4	---	72.5	218,000	1.7	7.8
1930------------------------	1,126,856	9.2	---	67.2	195,961	1.6	7.5

[1]Estimated for 1935, 1955, 1960, and 1965-69.
[2]Estimated. Reported annulments included.

VI. HEALTH CHARACTERISTICS

The Division of Health Interview Statistics obtains data on a wide variety of health topics. These data are reported from household interviews conducted during each year in about 40,000 households consisting of about 116,000 persons. Data in tables 12 and 13 are based on interviews during 1975, while data in table 14 are based on data collected during 1974. The data refer to the civilian, noninstitutional population of the United States. During 1975 this population averaged 209,065,000 persons. In 1974 this population averaged 207,344,000.

Table 12. Selected health statistics: 1975

Health topic	Estimated national annual frequency
Number of acute conditions:[1]	
Infective and parasitic diseases	47,608,000
Common cold	93,305,000
Other acute respiratory conditions	139,655,000
Acute digestive conditions	21,618,000
Injuries	76,192,000
All other acute conditions	64,741,000
Number of days of disability:[2]	
Restricted-activity days	3,733,892,000
Bed days	1,371,418,000
School-loss days (ages 6-16 years)	217,102,000
Work-loss days (reported for currently employed persons 17 years and over)	433,152,000
Number of persons with limited activity due to chronic disease or impairment:	
With any degree of limitation of activity	29,900,000
With limitations in major activity[3]	22,519,000
Medical and dental care:	
Number of physician visits	1,056,094,000
Home visits	8,217,000
Office visits	717,746,000
Other visits or consultations	330,131,000
Number of dental visits	340,882,000
Number of persons injured:[4]	
In moving motor vehicle accidents	5,140,000
In work accidents	9,841,000
In home accidents	31,197,000
In all other accidents	28,352,000

[1]Includes only acute conditions for which a doctor was consulted or which caused the person to restrict his normal daily activities for at least 1 day.

[2]Not mutually exclusive. A work- or school-loss day may also be a bed day. Work-loss days, school-loss days, and bed days are included in restricted-activity days.

[3]Refers to ability to work, keep house, or engage in school or preschool activities.

[4]Includes only persons whose injuries required medical attention or resulted in at least 1 day of activity restriction. The classes of accidents are not mutually exclusive, e.g., a person injured in a moving motor vehicle while at work is classified in both categories.

Table 13. Leading causes of bed disability due to acute conditions: 1975

[Data are based on household interviews of the civilian, noninstitutionalized population]

Cause	Number in thousands	Percent
All acute conditions	866,374	100.0
Respiratory conditions	429,549	49.6
Influenza	231,759	26.8
Cold and other upper respiratory conditions	142,706	16.5
Pneumonia, bronchitis, and other acute lower respiratory conditions	55,084	6.4
Injuries	141,906	16.4
Fractures, dislocations, sprains and strains	73,413	8.5
Infective and parasitic diseases	99,780	11.5
Virus, N.O.S.	36,814	4.2
Common childhood diseases	13,892	1.6
Digestive system conditions	48,442	5.6
Genitourinary disorders	24,142	2.8
Deliveries and disorders of pregnancy and the puerperium	26,067	3.0
Diseases of the ear	19,284	2.2
Diseases of the musculoskeletal system	19,746	2.3
All other acute conditions	57,457	6.6

In general, the items listed follow commonly accepted definitions. Technical aspects of the data and more detailed information about the topics are given in the report entitled "Health Survey Procedure" (*Vital and Health Statistics,* Series 1, No. 2).

The Division of Health Interview Statistics obtains data on chronic conditions reported to have caused or contributed to limitation of activities. The estimates shown in table 14 include conditions limiting major activities such as working, keeping house, and going to school as well as those causing lesser limitation not related to major activity. Excluded are conditions causing limitation among persons in resident institutions, sanitariums, chronic disease hospitals, nursing homes, and homes for the aged.

Additional data about conditions causing limitation of activities are shown in "Limitation of Activity Due to Chronic Conditions" (*Vital and Health Statistics,* Series 10, No. 111).

Table 14. Number of persons with limitation of activity by selected chronic conditions causing limitation: 1974

[Data are based on household interviews of the civilian noninstitutionalized population]

Condition causing limitation of activity	Number of persons[1]
Persons limited in activity	29,292,000
Tuberculosis, all forms	122,000
Malignant neoplasms	633,000
Benign and unspecified neoplasms	262,000
Diabetes	1,448,000
Mental and nervous conditions	1,504,000
Heart conditions	4,753,000
Cerebrovascular disease	793,000
Hypertension without heart involvement	1,976,000
Varicose veins	267,000
Hemorrhoids	92,000
Other conditions of circulatory system	1,148,000
Chronic bronchitis	293,000
Emphysema	822,000
Asthma, with or without hay fever	1,434,000
Hay fever, without asthma	210,000
Chronic sinusitis	191,000
Other conditions of respiratory system	602,000
Peptic ulcer	550,000
Hernia	690,000
Other conditions of digestive system	948,000
Diseases of kidney and ureter	358,000
Other conditions of genitourinary system	488,000
Arthritis and rheumatism	4,396,000
Other musculoskeletal disorders	1,718,000
Visual impairments	1,724,000
Hearing impairments	702,000
Paralysis, complete or partial	974,000
Impairments (except paralysis) of back or spine	2,051,000
Impairments (except paralysis and absence) of upper extremities and shoulders	650,000
Impairments (except paralysis and absence) of lower extremities and hips	1,889,000

[1]Summations of conditions causing limitation may be greater than the number of persons limited because a person can report more than one condition as a cause of his limitation; on the other hand, they may be less because only selected conditions are shown.

13

Table 15. Communicable diseases—reported cases and registered deaths: 1969-76

[Numbers after diseases are category numbers of the Eighth Revision International Classification of Diseases, Adapted, 1965. Since frequencies are for calendar years, not all deaths necessarily resulted from the cases tallied]

Diseases	1976	1975	1974	1973	1972[1]	1971	1970	1969
Amebiasis (006):								
Cases ------------	2,906	2,775	2,743	2,235	2,199	2,752	2,888	2,915
Deaths -----------	36	35	25	31	52	60	59	58
Anthrax (022):								
Cases ------------	2	2	2	2	2	5	2	4
Deaths -----------	-	-	-	-	-	-	-	-
Botulism (005.1):								
Cases ------------	37	17	28	34	22	25	12	16
Deaths -----------	3	3	6	6	6	7	7	4
Brucellosis (undulant fever) (023):								
Cases ------------	296	310	240	202	196	183	213	235
Deaths -----------	2	-	-	1	6	3	2	3
Diphtheria (032):								
Cases ------------	128	307	272	228	152	215	435	241
Deaths -----------	7	5	5	10	10	13	30	25
Dysentery, bacillary (004):								
Cases ------------	13,140	16,584	22,600	22,642	20,207	16,143	13,845	11,946
Deaths -----------	19	27	32	33	38	24	30	36
Encephalitis, acute infectious (062-065,079.2):								
Cases ------------	1,518	3,815	1,066	1,618	1,059	1,524	1,580	1,613
Deaths -----------	253	386	276	326	266	320	327	386
Hepatitis, infectious (070):								
Cases ------------	33,288	35,855	40,358	50,749	54,074	59,606	56,797	48,416
Deaths -----------	567	612	630	656	778	906	1,014	1,011
Leprosy (030):								
Cases ------------	145	162	118	146	130	131	129	98
Deaths -----------	1	2	2	1	-	1	5	4
Malaria (084):								
Cases ------------	471	373	293	237	742	2,375	3,051	3,102
Deaths -----------	4	4	4	7	-	6	5	11
Measles (055):								
Cases ------------	41,126	24,374	22,094	26,690	32,275	75,290	47,351	25,826
Deaths -----------	12	20	20	23	24	90	89	41
Meningococcal infections (036):								
Cases ------------	1,605	1,478	1,346	1,378	1,323	2,262	2,505	2,951
Deaths -----------	330	308	305	330	350	509	550	744
Plague (020):								
Cases ------------	16	20	8	2	1	2	13	5
Deaths -----------	2	3	1	-	-	-	1	-
Poliomyelitis, acute (040,041,043):								
Cases ------------	14	8	7	8	31	21	33	20
Paralytic -------	12	8	7	7	29	17	31	18
Deaths[2] ----------	16	9	3	10	2	18	7	13
Psittacosis (073):								
Cases ------------	78	49	164	33	52	32	35	57
Deaths -----------	-	-	-	1	-	1	1	-

ν

Table 15. Communicable diseases—reported cases and registered deaths: 1969-76—Con.

[Numbers after diseases are category numbers of the Eighth Revision International Classification of Diseases, Adapted, 1965. Since frequencies are for calendar years, not all deaths necessarily resulted from the cases tallied]

Diseases	1976	1975	1974	1973	1972[1]	1971	1970	1969
Rabies in man (071):								
Cases-----------	2	2	-	1	2	2	2	1
Deaths----------	1	2	-	1	2	2	2	1
Rocky Mountain spotted fever (082.0):								
Cases-----------	937	844	754	668	523	432	380	498
Deaths----------	41	29	49	38	50	36	29	36
Rubella (German measles) (056):								
Cases-----------	12,491	16,652	11,917	27,804	25,507	45,086	56,552	57,686
Deaths----------	12	21	15	16	14	20	31	29
Salmonellosis, excl. typhoid fever (002,003):								
Cases-----------	22,937	22,612	21,980	23,818	22,151	21,928	22,096	18,419
Deaths[3]----------	61	67	59	76	68	81	81	82
Tetanus (037):								
Cases-----------	75	102	101	101	128	116	148	185
Deaths----------	32	45	44	40	58	64	79	89
Trichinosis (124):								
Cases-----------	115	252	120	102	89	103	109	222
Deaths----------	1	-	-	1	2	4	1	-
Tuberculosis, all forms (010-019):								
Cases[4]-----------	32,105	33,989	30,122	30,998	32,882	35,217	37,137	39,120
Deaths----------	3,130	3,333	3,513	3,875	4,376	4,501	5,217	5,567
Tularemia (021):								
Cases-----------	157	129	144	171	152	187	172	149
Deaths----------	2	-	2	4	-	2	2	1
Typhoid fever (001):								
Cases-----------	419	375	437	680	398	407	346	364
Deaths----------	2	3	3	7	8	4	6	4
Typhus fever, endemic (081.0):								
Cases-----------	69	44	26	32	18	23	27	36
Deaths----------	1	-	-	1	-	-	-	-
Whooping cough (033):								
Cases-----------	1,010	1,738	2,402	1,759	3,287	3,036	4,249	3,285
Deaths----------	7	8	14	5	6	18	12	13
Venereal diseases[5]								
Gonorrhea (098):								
Cases-----------	1,001,994	999,937	898,943	842,621	767,215	670,268	600,072	534,872
Deaths----------	1	1	1	11	8	9	9	3
Syphilis (090-097):								
Cases-----------	71,761	80,356	83,771	87,469	91,149	95,997	91,382	92,162
Deaths----------	225	272	300	393	344	375	461	543

[1]Deaths based on a 50-percent sample.
[2]Excludes late effects of acute poliomyelitis.
[3]Including paratyphoid fever.
[4]New diagnostic standards introduced in 1975.
[5]Newly reported civilian cases.

SOURCE: Reported cases of communicable diseases came from the Center for Disease Control, Public Health Service, Atlanta, Ga.

The Division of Health Examination Statistics obtains data on the prevalence of selected chronic conditions and physical measurements of the U.S. population by direct examinations of persons selected in national probability samples. Tables 18 and 19 are based on data collected on adults in 1960-1962. Table 17 presents data on children aged 6-11 years collected in 1963-1965, while tables 16 and 20 additionally present data on youths aged 6-17 collected in 1966-1970.

Additional data on adults, children, and youth are presented in the more than 75 reports in Series 11 of *Vital and Health Statistics*.

Table 16. Dental, sensory, and speech defects in youths aged 12-17 years: 1966-70

Condition and sex	Total	Age in years					
		12	13	14	15	16	17
Filled teeth per youth[1]	3.8	2.3	2.8	3.5	4.2	4.6	5.6
Boys, average	3.5	2.1	2.6	3.1	4.0	4.2	5.2
Girls, average	4.1	2.6	3.0	3.8	4.5	5.1	6.0
Decayed teeth per youth[1]	1.7	1.2	1.5	1.8	1.9	1.9	2.0
Boys, average	1.7	1.2	1.3	1.8	1.8	1.9	2.2
Girls, average	1.7	1.3	1.6	1.7	2.0	1.8	1.8
Defective visual acuity uncorrected[2]							
Rate per 100 youths	22.4	18.6	23.1	22.7	21.5	25.0	24.2
Boys	19.1	15.6	17.4	18.2	20.8	22.8	19.6
Girls	26.0	21.8	28.8	27.2	22.2	27.4	28.7
Defective visual acuity with usual correction[3]							
Rate per 100 youths	5.0	6.0	6.6	5.6	4.6	3.1	3.0
Boys	3.9	4.0	5.6	4.6	3.4	2.9	2.4
Girls	5.9	8.3	7.5	6.6	5.6	3.2	3.3
Defective hearing[4]							
Rate per 100 youths	0.7	0.8	0.8	0.5	0.5	0.9	0.7
Boys	0.9	1.1	0.8	0.6	0.5	1.3	1.1
Girls	0.5	0.6	0.9	0.4	0.7	0.4	0.2
Speech defects or trouble talking[5]							
Rate per 100 youths	4.3	4.9	5.8	3.6	4.0	3.7	3.6
Boys	5.2	5.1	7.3	4.6	5.4	4.6	4.1
Girls	3.3	4.7	4.2	2.5	2.7	2.8	3.1

[1]Average number per youth.
[2]Binocular visual acuity of 20/40 or less (Snellen ratio) without correction.
[3]Binocular visual acuity of 20/40 or less (Snellen ratio) with own glasses, if worn, or without correction if youth does not wear glasses.
[4]Hearing levels in better ear of 16 decibels or more above audiometric zero (ASA, 1951) at frequencies essential for speech (500, 1000, and 2000 Hertz).
[5]Report from parent.

SOURCE: National Center for Health Statistics, Series 11, Nos. 127, 129, 144, and 145, Vital and Health Statistics.

Table 17. Dental, sensory, and speech defects in children aged 6-11 years: 1963-65

Condition and sex	Total	Age in years					
		6	7	8	9	10	11
Filled primary teeth per child[1]	1.2	1.2	1.4	1.6	1.4	1.0	0.5
Boys, average	1.3	1.1	1.4	1.7	1.4	1.2	0.6
Girls, average	1.1	1.2	1.3	1.6	1.4	0.9	0.4
Filled permanent teeth per child	0.8	0.1	0.2	0.6	1.0	1.4	1.6
Boys, average	0.7	0.1	0.2	0.5	0.8	1.4	1.4
Girls, average	0.9	0.1	0.3	0.7	1.1	1.4	1.9
Decayed primary teeth per child[1]	1.4	2.0	2.0	1.8	1.4	1.0	0.5
Boys, average	1.5	1.9	2.0	1.8	1.6	1.0	0.6
Girls, average	1.4	2.0	2.0	1.7	1.3	0.9	0.4
Decayed permanent teeth per child[1]	0.4	0.1	0.3	0.4	0.6	0.7	0.8
Boys, average	0.4	0.1	0.2	0.4	0.6	0.7	0.7
Girls, average	0.5	0.1	0.4	0.4	0.6	0.7	1.0
<u>Defective visual acuity uncorrected[2]</u>							
Rate per 100 children	11.1	7.4	9.3	9.1	10.2	13.4	17.2
Boys	10.3	6.6	9.1	9.4	9.1	11.6	16.1
Girls	11.9	8.3	9.5	9.0	11.5	15.3	18.3
<u>Defective hearing[3]</u>							
Rate per 100 children	0.5	0.1	0.5	0.7	1.0	0.4	0.5
Boys	0.5	0.2	0.8	0.9	0.8	0.2	0.5
Girls	0.4	-	0.2	0.5	1.2	0.7	0.5
<u>Speech defects or problems talking[4]</u>							
Rate per 100 children	8.4	12.8	9.6	7.5	7.1	6.8	6.2
Boys	9.9	14.8	11.2	8.8	8.6	8.4	7.4
Girls	6.8	10.9	7.9	6.1	5.5	5.1	4.9

[1]Average number per child.
[2]Binocular visual acuity of 20/40 or less (Snellen ratio) without correction.
[3]Hearing levels in the better ear of 16 decibels or more above audiometric zero (ASA, 1951) at frequencies essential for speech (500, 1000, and 2000 Hertz).
[4]Report from parent.

SOURCE: National Center for Health Statistics. Series 11, Nos. 101, 102, 106, and 108, <u>Vital and Health Statistics</u>.

Table 18. Prevalence rates of heart disease, hypertension, and arthritis in adults by age and sex: 1960-62

[Rates per 100 persons in specified group]

Diagnosis and sex	Total	Age group in years						
		18-24	25-34	35-44	45-54	55-64	65-74	75-79
Definite heart disease, total[1]								
Both sexes	13.2	1.2	2.4	6.7	13.2	25.3	39.9	42.3
Men	12.6	1.4	2.9	7.4	13.8	24.2	33.2	38.8
Women	13.7	1.1	2.0	6.1	12.5	26.2	45.2	45.8
Suspect heart disease, total[1]								
Both sexes	11.7	4.0	4.9	8.8	15.3	19.4	20.7	25.2
Men	13.9	6.4	6.6	11.4	18.3	18.5	25.3	27.1
Women	9.7	2.0	3.3	6.4	12.4	20.1	17.1	23.3
Definite hypertensive heart disease								
Both sexes	9.5	0.3	1.3	4.7	9.6	17.9	30.3	31.8
Men	7.7	0.4	1.4	5.2	9.7	13.6	18.9	24.6
Women	11.1	0.2	1.2	4.2	9.5	21.9	39.5	39.0
Suspect hypertensive heart disease								
Both sexes	4.3	0.7	1.1	2.6	4.4	8.4	10.4	14.1
Men	5.1	1.5	1.7	4.2	5.0	7.8	12.8	16.1
Women	3.5	-	0.6	1.1	3.8	9.0	8.5	12.1
Definite coronary heart disease								
Both sexes	2.8	-	0.3	0.7	2.5	7.1	9.5	6.8
Men	3.7	-	0.4	1.1	3.5	9.7	11.6	9.1
Women	2.0	-	0.2	0.5	1.6	4.7	7.9	4.5
Suspect coronary heart disease								
Both sexes	2.2	-	0.1	0.9	3.0	4.8	5.9	5.7
Men	2.2	-	-	1.3	3.4	4.4	5.3	3.8
Women	2.2	-	0.2	0.5	2.5	5.2	6.4	7.5
Definite hypertension								
Both sexes	15.3	1.4	3.9	10.9	18.2	26.9	38.5	38.8
Men	14.1	1.7	4.8	13.5	18.3	22.3	27.1	32.4
Women	16.4	1.2	3.1	8.5	18.2	31.2	47.6	45.1
Borderline hypertension								
Both sexes	14.6	5.7	7.4	11.5	16.5	25.9	24.5	27.5
Men	17.2	10.9	11.9	14.2	17.7	27.5	24.8	26.7
Women	12.2	1.4	3.2	9.0	15.3	24.5	24.3	28.3
Rheumatoid arthritis								
Both sexes	3.2	0.3	0.3	1.3	3.0	6.3	9.2	18.8
Men	1.7	0.2	-	0.5	1.5	4.2	3.1	14.1
Women	4.6	0.3	0.6	2.1	4.4	8.3	14.1	23.5
Osteoarthritis								
Both sexes	37.4	4.1	9.7	24.7	46.6	69.4	80.7	85.4
Men	37.4	7.2	13.6	30.2	47.0	63.2	75.8	80.9
Women	37.3	1.6	6.2	19.6	46.3	75.2	84.7	89.8

[1]Includes persons with other types of heart disease not shown separately.

18

VII. PHYSICAL MEASUREMENTS

Table 19. Weight range of men and women by age and height: 1960-62

[Height in feet and inches, without shoes; weight in pounds, partially clothed. Clothing weight estimated at 2 lb. Values shown represent range of weights within which 50 percent of the population of a given height would fall. Approximately 25 percent would weigh less and 25 percent more than these values]

Height and sex	Weight by age group in years						
	18-24	25-34	35-44	45-54	55-64	65-74	75-79
Men							
5'2"------------------------	120-154	121-161	131-167	130-167	128-168	125-163	116-151
5'3"------------------------	123-157	126-165	134-170	134-171	131-171	128-167	121-156
5'4"------------------------	127-161	130-170	138-174	138-175	135-175	132-170	126-161
5'5"------------------------	130-164	135-174	142-178	142-179	138-178	135-174	131-166
5'6"------------------------	134-168	139-178	146-182	146-183	142-182	138-177	136-171
5'7"------------------------	137-171	144-183	150-186	150-187	146-186	142-180	142-176
5'8"------------------------	141-175	148-187	153-189	154-191	149-189	145-184	146-181
5'9"------------------------	144-178	153-192	157-193	158-195	153-193	149-187	151-186
5'10"-----------------------	148-182	157-196	161-197	162-199	156-196	152-191	156-191
5'11"-----------------------	151-185	162-201	164-200	166-203	160-200	156-194	162-196
6'--------------------------	155-189	166-205	168-204	170-207	163-204	159-198	167-201
6'1"------------------------	158-192	170-210	172-208	174-211	167-207	162-201	172-206
6'2"------------------------	162-196	175-214	176-212	178-215	171-211	166-204	177-212
Women							
4'9"------------------------	98-133	90-133	109-153	107-151	116-160	112-151	106-145
4'10"-----------------------	100-135	94-137	111-156	110-154	119-163	116-154	109-149
4'11"-----------------------	103-138	98-141	114-158	114-158	122-166	119-158	113-152
5'--------------------------	105-140	102-145	116-160	118-161	125-169	123-161	116-156
5'1"------------------------	107-142	106-149	118-162	121-165	128-171	126-164	120-159
5'2"------------------------	110-144	110-153	120-165	125-169	131-174	130-168	123-163
5'3"------------------------	112-146	114-157	123-167	128-172	134-177	133-171	126-166
5'4"------------------------	114-149	118-161	125-169	132-176	136-180	137-175	130-170
5'5"------------------------	116-151	122-165	127-172	136-179	139-183	140-178	133-173
5'6"------------------------	118-153	126-169	129-174	139-183	142-186	144-182	137-176
5'7"------------------------	121-155	130-173	132-176	143-187	145-189	147-185	140-180
5'8"------------------------	123-158	134-177	134-178	146-190	148-191	150-189	144-183

Table 20. Weight range of boys and girls 6-17

[Height in inches, without shoes; weight in pounds, partially clothed. Values given height and age would fall. Approximately 25 percent would weigh

	Sex and height in inches	6 years	7 years	8 years
	Girls		Interquartile range of	
1	Under 41.3---	35-39		
2	41.3-43.2---	40-45		
3	43.3-45.2---	43-49	40-44	
4	45.3-47.2---	48-54	43-49	43-52
5	47.3-49.1---	52-62	48-55	46-54
6	49.2-51.1---		52-63	52-62
7	51.2-53.1---		56-65	58-67
8	53.2-55.1---			64-77
9	55.2-57.0---			75-93
10	57.1-59.0---			
11	59.1-61.0---			
12	61.1-63.0---			
13	63.1-65.0---			
14	65.1-66.9---			
15	67.0-68.9---			
16	69.0-70.9---			
	Boys			
17	41.3-43.2---	37-41		
18	43.3-45.2---	40-45	41-46	
19	45.3-47.2---	44-50	44-50	43-49
20	47.3-49.1---	48-55	48-54	49-54
21	49.2-51.1---	53-60	53-60	53-60
22	51.2-53.1---		57-66	59-67
23	53.2-55.1---		63-71	64-76
24	55.2-57.0---			69-77
25	57.1-59.0---			
26	59.1-61.0---			
27	61.1-63.0---			
28	63.1-65.0---			
29	65.1-66.9---			
30	67.0-68.9---			
31	69.0-70.9---			
32	71.0-72.8---			
33	72.9-74.8---			
34	74.9-76.8---			

[1] The middle 50 percent of the weight range (P_{75} - P_{25}).

years of age by single year of age and height: 1963-70

shown represent range of weight within which 50 percent of children of
less and 25 percent more than these values]

weight in pounds[1]

9 years	10 years	11 years	12 years	13 years	14 years	15 years	16 years	17 years	
									1
									2
									3
									4
49-56									5
53-62	52-58								6
57-66	57-65	60-69							7
64-77	62-77	64-78	58-71						8
71-89	71-81	69-82	73-91	67-88					9
73-102	78-94	76-94	78-94	84-97	80-105	93-116	99-120	88-101	10
	82-99	84-106	86-104	86-104	94-118	98-116	101-119	98-118	11
		94-122	95-119	97-119	102-123	102-122	107-124	107-127	12
		102-134	104-126	105-126	107-132	111-133	114-135	111-127	13
			111-132	115-136	115-136	122-145	118-148	122-144	14
			112-181	107-144	124-155	126-158	128-147	122-145	15
					127-142	119-156	136-178	132-166	16
									17
									18
									19
49-54									20
53-61									21
58-65	55-61	61-71							22
63-74	58-66	65-75							23
70-83	64-74	71-82	67-76	64-77					24
71-103	70-80	77-91	70-80	71-86	87-93				25
	77-92	83-101	79-90	80-91	86-106	94-101			26
	81-95	94-120	84-101	84-100	92-113	103-125	98-120	106-127	27
			92-111	92-113	105-124	103-124	106-128	116-136	28
			99-123	103-128	114-137	117-135	116-141	124-148	29
			108-132	109-131	121-145	125-148	127-148	131-158	30
			132-146	118-148	129-154	132-153	134-160	136-162	31
				132-155	144-170	142-173	142-169	144-173	32
						139-186	154-199	155-178	33
						153-227	*	150-199	34

21

VIII. HEALTH RESOURCES

Table 21. Estimated persons employed in selected occupations within each health field: 1974

Health field and occupation	Active workers
Total[1]	4,672,850 to 4,707,650
Administration of health services	[2]48,200
Health department, public health administrator	5,200
Hospital administrator and assistant	17,000
Nursing home administrator and assistant	16,000
Voluntary health agency administrator and program representative	10,000
Anthropology and sociology	1,700
Anthropologist—cultural and physical	[2]700
Sociologist—medical	1,000
Automatic data processing in the health field	4,000 to 5,000
Systems analyst and programer	4,000 to 5,000
Basic sciences in the health field[3]	60,000
Research scientist (other than physician, dentist, veterinarian)	60,000
Biomedical engineering	12,000
Biomedical engineer	4,000
Biomedical engineering technician	8,000
Chiropractic	16,600
Chiropractor	16,600
Clinical laboratory services	172,500
Clinical laboratory scientist	5,500
Clinical laboratory technologist	97,000
Clinical laboratory technician and assistant	70,000
Dentistry and allied services	279,800
Dentist	107,300
Dental hygienist	22,500
Dental assistant	118,000
Dental laboratory technician	32,000
Dietetic and nutritional services	72,700
Dietitian and nutritionist	48,000
Dietetic technician and food service supervisor	24,700
Economic research in the health field	[2]400
Economist—health	400

See footnotes at end of table.

Table 21. Estimated persons employed in selected occupations within each health field: 1974—Con.

Health field and occupation	Active workers
Environmental sanitation	20,000
Sanitarian	15,000
Technician and aide	5,000
Food and drug protective services	47,900
Inspector (health, food and drug, other)	16,400
Food and drug chemist or microbiologist	1,100
Food technologist	27,000
Food technician	[2]3,400
Funeral directing and embalming	50,000
Funeral director and embalmer	50,000
Health and vital statistics	[4]1,350
Health statistician	1,100
Vital record registrar	150
Demographer	100
Health education	22,500 to 23,000
Public health educator	2,500 to 3,000
School health educator or coordinator	[2]20,000
Health information and communication	7,400 to 10,500
Biomedical photographer	2,000 to 3,000
Health information specialist and science writer	2,000 to 4,000
Medical writer	1,400
Technical writer and editor	1,500
Medical illustrator	[2]500 to 600
Library services in the health field	10,300
Medical librarian	3,000
Medical library technician and clerk	7,300
Medical records	60,000
Registered record administrator	5,500
Accredited record technician	7,500
Other medical record personnel	47,000
Medicine and osteopathy	362,700
Physician (M.D.)	350,600
Physician (D.O.)	12,100

See footnotes at end of table.

Table 21. Estimated persons employed in selected occupations within each health field: 1974—Con.

Health field and occupation	Active workers
Midwifery	4,300
Lay midwife	2,500
Nurse-midwife	1,800
Nursing and related services	2,319,000
Registered nurse	857,000
Practical nurse	492,000
Nursing aide, orderly or attendant	936,000
Home health aide	34,000
Occupational therapy	13,500 to 14,500
Occupational therapist	8,000
Occupational therapy technician or assistant	[2]5,500 to 6,500
Opticianry	12,000
Dispensing optician	12,000
Optometry	25,100 to 25,300
Optometrist	19,300
Optometric assistant	[2]5,000
Optometric technician	[2]800 to 1,000
Orthotic and prosthetic technology	2,800 to 3,800
Orthotist and prosthetist	2,800 to 3,800
Pharmacy	132,900
Pharmacist	132,900
Physical therapy	26,100
Physical therapist	18,000
Physical therapy technician or assistant	8,100
Podiatric medicine	7,100
Podiatrist	7,100
Psychology	35,000
Psychologist	35,000
Radiologic technology	100,000
Radiologic (X-ray) technologist, technician or assistant	100,000

See footnotes at end of table.

Table 21. Estimated persons employed in selected occupations within each health field: 1974—Con.

Health field and occupation	Active workers
Respiratory therapy	18,000 to 19,000
Respiratory therapist and technician	18,000 to 19,000
Secretarial and office services in the health field	[2]275,000 to 300,000
Receptionist, secretary, assistant, or aide	275,000 to 300,000
Social work	38,600
Social worker—medical and psychiatric	34,300
Social work assistant and aide	[4]4,300
Specialized rehabilitation services	11,250 to 13,250
Corrective therapist	1,100
Educational therapist	400
Manual arts therapist	1,000
Music therapist	2,200
Therapeutic recreational specialist	6,000 to 8,000
Home economist in rehabilitation	550
Speech pathology and audiology	27,000
Speech pathologist and audiologist	27,000
Veterinary medicine	33,500
Veterinarian	28,500
Animal technician	5,000
Vocational rehabilitation counseling	17,700
Vocational rehabilitation counselor	17,700
Miscellaneous health services	323,950
Electrocardiograph technician	[2]9,500
Electroencephalograph technician	4,000
Emergency medical technician	260,000
Medical assistant	16,000
Operating room technician	12,000
Ophthalmic medical assistant	20,000
Orthoptist	[2]450
Physician's assistant	2,000

[1]Each occupation is counted only once. For example, all physicians are in medicine and osteopathy.
[2]Previous estimate repeated in absence of sufficient information on which to base revision.
[3]Statistics are not available on what percentage of the estimated 250,000 physical scientists are employed in the health field.
[4]1968 estimate repeated in absence of sufficient information on which to base revision.

SOURCE: National Center for Health Statistics: Health Resources Statistics, 1975, Pub. No.(HRA) 76-1509. Health Resources Administration, Washington. U.S. Government Printing Office, 1976.

Table 22. Physicians in relation to population: Selected years, 1950-76

Year	Population in thousands	Number of physicians			Physicians per 100,000 population
		M.D. and D.O.[1]	M.D.[2]	D.O.[1]	
	Total[3]	All physicians, active and inactive			
1976--	219,370	425,016	409,446	15,570	194
1975--	217,829	409,042	393,742	15,300	188
1974--	216,304	394,448	379,748	14,700	182
1973--	214,583	380,679	366,379	14,300	177
1972--	213,046	370,534	356,534	14,000	174
1971--	211,578	---	344,823	---	---
1970--	209,539	---	334,028	---	---
1969--	207,863	---	324,942	---	---
1968--	205,758	---	317,032	---	---
1965--	199,278	305,115	292,088	13,027	153
1960--	185,370	274,833	260,484	14,349	148
1955--	170,499	255,211	241,711	13,500	150
1950--	156,472	232,697	219,997	12,700	149
	Total[3]	All active non-Federal and Federal physicians[4]			
1976--	219,370	---	378,572	---	---
1975--	217,829	---	366,425	---	---
1974--	216,304	---	350,609	---	---
1973--	214,583	---	338,111	---	---
1972--	213,046	---	333,259	---	---
1971--	211,578	---	322,228	---	---
1970--	209,539	---	311,203	---	---
1969--	207,863	---	302,966	---	---
1968--	205,758	---	296,312	---	---
1965--	199,278	288,671	277,575	11,096	145
1960--	185,370	259,420	247,257	12,163	140
1955--	170,499	240,153	228,553	11,600	141
1950--	156,472	219,897	208,997	10,900	141
	Civilian	Non-Federal physicians providing patient care[5]			
1976--	216,267	---	294,730	---	---
1975--	214,735	---	287,837	---	---
1974--	213,219	---	278,517	---	---
1973--	211,507	---	272,850	---	---
1972--	209,979	---	269,095	---	---
1971--	208,691	273,861	263,730	10,131	131
1970--	206,093	---	255,027	---	---
1969--	203,989	---	247,508	---	---
1968--	201,787	---	238,481	---	---

Table 22. Physicians in relation to population: Selected years, 1950-76—Con.

| Year | Population in thousands | Number of physicians | | | Physicians per 100,000 population |
| | | M.D. and D.O.[1] | M.D.[2] | D.O.[1] | |
	Civilian	Non-Federal physicians providing patient care in office-based practice			
1976	216,267	---	214,710	---	---
1975	214,735	---	213,334	---	---
1974	213,219	---	203,943	---	---
1973	211,507	---	199,134	---	---
1972	209,979	---	198,974	---	---
1971	208,691	203,748	194,932	8,816	98
1970	206,093	---	188,924	---	---
1969	203,989	---	184,355	---	---
1968	201,787	---	180,991	---	---

[1]Estimated.

[2]Includes non-Federal physicians in 50 States, District of Columbia, Puerto Rico, and other U.S. outlying areas (American Samoa, Canal Zone, Guam, Pacific Islands, and Virgin Islands), those with addresses temporarily unknown to American Medical Association; and Federal physicians in the United States and abroad. Excludes physicians with temporary foreign addresses.

[3]Includes civilians in 50 States, District of Columbia, Puerto Rico, and other U.S. outlying areas; U.S. citizens in foreign countries; and the Armed Forces in the United States and abroad.

[4]Excludes physicians with addresses temporarily unknown to the American Medical Association and those whose status was not reported to the American Osteopathic Association. Includes for 1970-1976 M.D.'s not classified as to their specialty or activity.

[5]Includes physicians in solo practice and in partnership, group, or other forms of office practice and those in hospital-based practice—interns, residents, fellows, and full-time hospital staff.

SOURCES: Goodman, Louis J., and Mason, Henry R.: Physician Distribution and Medical Licensure in the U.S., 1975. Chicago. AMA Center for Health Services Research and Development, American Medical Association, 1976.

Divisions of Public Health Methods, Dental Public Health and Resources, and Nursing; Manpower in the 1960's. Health Manpower Source Book 18. PHS Pub. No. 263, Section 18. Public Health Service, U.S. Department of Health, Education, and Welfare. Washington. U.S. Government Printing Office, 1964, table 12.

U.S. Bureau of the Census: Current Population Reports. Series P-25, No. 703. Also, prior reports, 1970 Census of Population including Series PC(1), Nos. 53 and 55. Also, unpublished estimates.

Table 23. Physicians by type of practice: Selected years, 1968-74

Type of practice	M.D.[1]			D.O.[2]
	1974	1970	1968	1971
Total	379,748	334,028	317,032	10,903
Active physicians	350,609	311,203	296,312	10,067
Non-Federal	345,607	301,323	285,175	10,233
Patient care	278,517	255,027	238,481	8,373
Office-based practice	203,943	188,924	180,991	7,286
General practice[3]	50,201	53,257	54,994	5,460
Other full-time primary specialty	153,742	135,667	125,997	1,826
Hospital-based practice	74,574	66,103	57,490	1,087
Training programs[4]	54,510	45,840	41,545	883
Full-time hospital staff	20,064	20,263	15,945	204
Other professional activity[5]	25,133	26,317	28,063	195
Inactive	21,614	19,621	18,631	807
Not classified as to specialty	20,343	358	-	858
Federal	26,616	29,501	29,768	[6]670
Patient care	22,721	23,508	23,241	576
Office-based practice	2,012	3,515	3,623	382
General practice[3]	828	1,657	1,858	62
Other full-time primary specialty	1,184	1,858	1,765	320
Hospital-based practice	20,709	19,993	19,618	194
Training programs[4]	4,512	5,388	5,567	122
Full-time hospital staff	16,197	14,605	14,051	72
Other professional activity[5]	3,895	5,993	6,527	22
Address unknown	7,525	3,204	2,089	-

[1]Includes non-Federal physicians in the 50 States, District of Columbia, Puerto Rico, and other U.S. outlying areas (American Samoa, Canal Zone, Guam, Pacific Islands, and Virgin Islands); those with addresses temporarily unknown to the American Medical Association; and Federal physicians in the United States and abroad. Excludes physicians with temporary foreign addresses.
[2]Includes non-Federal and Federal physicians in the 50 States and the District of Columbia and those in U.S. possessions and foreign countries.
[3]Includes physicians reporting "no specialty" and specialties not listed on American Medical Association list of specialty designations.
[4]Includes interns and residents.
[5]Includes medical teaching, administration, research, and other activities.
[6]Includes 29 inactive physicians and 43 "not classified."

IX. MORTALITY

General

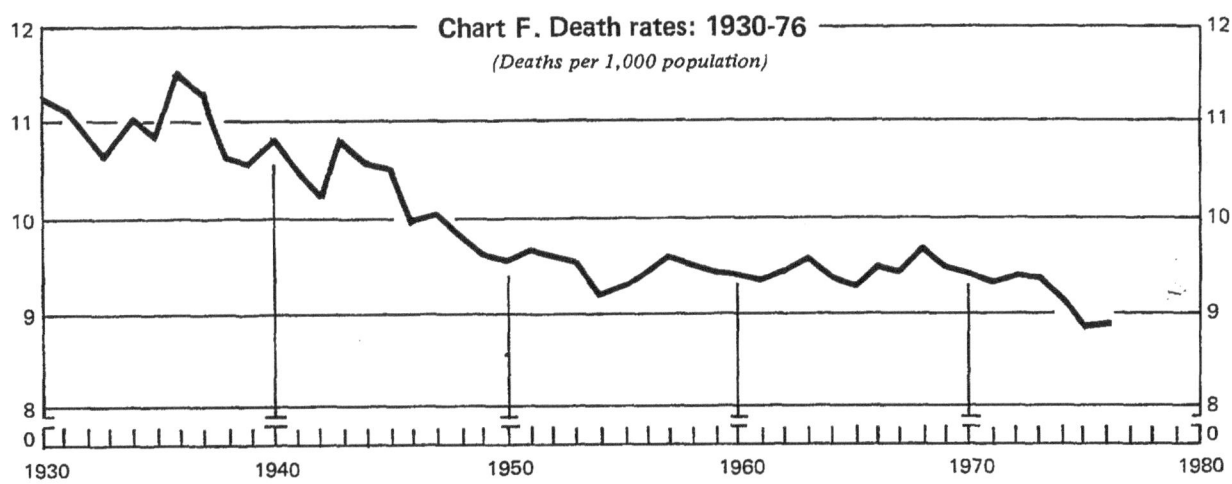

Chart F. Death rates: 1930-76

(Deaths per 1,000 population)

Table 24. Deaths, death rates, and age-adjusted death rates: Selected years, 1935-76

Year	Number	Rate per 1,000 population					Age-adjusted rate per 1,000 population[1]				
		Total	White		All other		Total	White		All other	
			Male	Female	Male	Female		Male	Female	Male	Female
1976[2]--------	1,909,440	8.9	10.1	7.9	9.8	6.8	6.3	8.0	4.4	10.7	6.4
1975[2]--------	1,892,879	8.9	10.2	7.8	10.0	6.8	6.4	8.1	4.5	11.0	6.5
1974[2]--------	1,934,388	9.2	10.4	8.1	10.4	7.2	6.7	8.4	4.7	11.5	6.9
1973[2]--------	1,973,003	9.4	10.7	8.2	10.8	7.6	6.9	8.7	4.8	12.1	7.4
1972[2,3]------	1,963,944	9.4	10.8	8.2	11.0	7.6	7.0	8.8	4.9	12.3	7.5
1971[2]--------	1,927,542	9.3	10.7	8.1	10.8	7.6	7.0	8.8	4.9	12.1	7.5
1970[2]--------	1,921,031	9.5	10.9	8.1	11.2	7.8	7.1	8.9	5.0	12.3	7.7
1969[4]--------	1,921,990	9.5	11.0	8.2	11.5	8.0	7.3	9.1	5.1	12.7	8.0
1968[4]--------	1,930,082	9.7	11.1	8.2	11.7	8.2	7.4	9.2	5.2	12.9	8.3
1967[4]--------	1,851,323	9.4	10.8	8.0	11.0	7.9	7.3	9.0	5.1	12.1	8.0
1966[4]--------	1,863,149	9.5	11.0	8.1	11.4	8.2	7.4	9.2	5.3	12.4	8.3
1965[4]--------	1,828,136	9.4	10.9	8.0	11.2	8.2	7.4	9.1	5.3	12.2	8.3
1960--------	1,711,982	9.5	11.0	8.0	11.5	8.7	7.6	9.2	5.6	12.1	8.9
1955--------	1,528,717	9.3	10.7	7.8	11.3	8.8	7.6	9.1	5.7	11.9	9.1
1950--------	1,452,454	9.6	10.9	8.0	12.5	9.9	8.4	9.6	6.5	13.6	11.0
1945--------	1,401,719	10.6	12.5	8.6	13.5	10.5	9.5	10.7	7.5	14.5	11.9
1940--------	1,417,269	10.8	11.6	9.2	15.1	12.6	10.8	11.6	8.8	17.6	15.0
1935--------	1,392,752	10.9	11.6	9.5	15.6	13.0	11.6	12.3	9.8	18.5	16.1

[1]Adjusted to age distribution of U.S. population as enumerated in 1940.
[2]Excludes deaths of nonresidents of the United States.
[3]Based on a 50-percent sample.
[4]Rates are revised.

Table 25. Deaths and death rates by age and sex: 1976

Age	Number			Rate per 1,000 population in specified group		
	Total	Male	Female	Total	Male	Female
All ages[1] -----------------------	1,909,440	1,051,983	857,457	8.9	10.1	7.8
Under 1 year----------------------------	48,265	27,320	20,945	16.0	17.6	14.2
1-4 years-------------------------------	8,606	4,915	3,691	0.7	0.8	0.6
5-9 years-------------------------------	6,034	3,626	2,408	0.3	0.4	0.3
10-14 years-----------------------------	6,867	4,442	2,425	0.3	0.4	0.3
15-19 years-----------------------------	20,561	15,001	5,560	1.0	1.4	0.5
20-24 years-----------------------------	25,520	19,252	6,268	1.3	2.0	0.6
25-29 years-----------------------------	22,902	16,431	6,471	1.3	1.9	0.7
30-34 years-----------------------------	20,527	13,731	6,796	1.4	2.0	0.9
35-39 years-----------------------------	23,555	15,106	8,449	2.0	2.6	1.4
40-44 years-----------------------------	34,914	22,054	12,860	3.1	4.1	2.3
45-49 years-----------------------------	58,061	36,746	21,315	5.0	6.5	3.6
50-54 years-----------------------------	91,975	58,578	33,397	7.7	10.2	5.4
55-59 years-----------------------------	126,361	80,982	45,379	11.8	15.8	8.1
60-64 years-----------------------------	169,699	108,713	60,986	18.2	25.0	12.3
65-69 years-----------------------------	210,465	131,351	79,114	25.4	35.9	17.1
70-74 years-----------------------------	233,462	136,115	97,347	39.5	54.3	28.6
75-79 years-----------------------------	250,623	131,056	119,567	61.9	82.6	48.5
80-84 years-----------------------------	246,096	113,137	132,959	90.3	115.2	76.3
85 years and over-----------------------	304,472	113,119	191,353	154.9	179.8	143.1

[1]Includes deaths for which age was not stated.

Leading Causes

The next table shows the number of deaths and death rates for the leading causes of death in 1976 and death rates for these causes in 1900.

Figures for the 2 years show gross changes in mortality, but they are not exactly comparable in many respects. The rates for 1900 are based on deaths in 10 States and the District of Columbia, while the figures for 1976 are for the entire United States. New discoveries in medicine and new diagnostic facilities have produced an improvement in reporting causes of death. Causes of death which were not recognized as disease entities in 1900 are relatively frequent in 1976. The classification of causes of death is revised every decade to keep abreast of new information.

For 1976 deaths were classified according to the Eighth Revision International Classification of Diseases, Adapted, and for 1900 according to the First Revision of the International Lists. Also, beginning with 1949, the underlying cause of death indicated by the physician is generally the cause used in statistical tabulation. In earlier years, a fixed set of priorities was used to select the cause of death to be tabulated when more than one cause was reported.

Table 26. Deaths and death rates for the 10 leading causes of death in 1976 and death rates for these same causes in 1900

Rank, 1976	Cause of death and category numbers of the Eighth Revision International Classification of Diseases, Adapted, 1965	Number of deaths, 1976	Rate per 100,000 population	
			1976	1900
	All causes--	1,909,440	889.6	1,719.1
1	Diseases of heart---------------------390-398,402,404,410-429	723,878	337.2	137.4
2	Malignant neoplasms, including neoplasms of lymphatic and hematopoietic tissues--------------------------------------140-209	377,312	175.8	64.0
3	Cerebrovascular diseases------------------------------------430-438	188,623	87.9	106.9
4	Accidents---E800-E949	100,761	46.9	72.3
5	Influenza and pneumonia-----------------------470-474,480-486	61,866	28.8	202.2
6	Diabetes mellitus---250	34,508	16.1	11.0
7	Cirrhosis of liver---571	31,453	14.7	12.5
8	Arteriosclerosis---440	29,366	13.7	---
9	Suicide--E950-E959	26,832	12.5	10.2
10	Certain causes of mortality in early infancy[1]-------------------------760,769.2,769.4-772,774-778	24,809	11.6	62.6

[1] Relates to birth injuries, asphyxia, infections of newborn, ill-defined diseases, immaturity, etc.

Table 27. Deaths and death rates for the 10 leading causes of death, by sex: 1976

Rank	Cause of death and category numbers of the Eighth Revision International Classification of Diseases, Adapted, 1965	Number	Rate per 100,000 population
	<u>Male</u>		
	All causes--	1,051,983	1,007.0
1	Diseases of heart----------------------------390-398,402,404,410-429	400,601	383.5
2	Malignant neoplasms, including neoplasms of lymphatic and		
	hematopoietic tissues---140-209	205,406	196.6
3	Cerebrovascular diseases---------------------------------------430-438	80,597	77.1
4	Accidents---E800-E949	70,277	67.3
5	Influenza and pneumonia----------------------------470-474,480-486	32,513	31.1
6	Cirrhosis of liver--571	20,668	19.8
7	Suicide---E950-E959	19,493	18.7
8	Bronchitis, emphysema, and asthma-------------------------490-493	17,784	17.0
9	Homicide--E960-E978	15,142	14.5
10	Certain causes of mortality in early		
	infancy--------------------------------760-769.2,769.4-772,774-778	14,198	13.6
	<u>Female</u>		
	All causes--	857,457	778.3
1	Diseases of heart----------------------------390-398,402,404,410-429	323,277	293.4
2	Malignant neoplasms, including neoplasms of lymphatic and		
	hematopoietic tissues---140-209	171,906	156.0
3	Cerebrovascular diseases---------------------------------------430-438	108,026	98.0
4	Accidents---E800-E949	30,484	27.7
5	Influenza and pneumonia----------------------------470-474,480-486	29,353	26.6
6	Diabetes mellitus---250	20,483	18.6
7	Arteriosclerosis--440	17,553	15.9
8	Cirrhosis of liver--571	10,785	9.8
9	Certain causes of mortality in early		
	infancy--------------------------------760-769.2,769.4-772,774-778	10,611	9.6
10	Suicide---E950-E959	7,339	6.7

Table 28. Deaths and death rates for the 10 leading causes of death in specified age and sex groups: 1976

Rank	Age, sex, cause of death, and category numbers of the Eighth Revision International Classification of Diseases, Adapted, 1965	Number	Rate per 100,000 population in specified group
	1-4 years, both sexes		
	All causes--	8,606	69.9
1	Accidents--E800-E949	3,439	27.9
2	Congenital anomalies--740-759	1,114	9.0
3	Malignant neoplasms, including neoplasms of lymphatic and hematopoietic tissues--------------------------------------140-209	656	5.3
4	Influenza and pneumonia-------------------------470-474,480-486	480	3.9
5	Homicide--E960-E978	306	2.5
6	Diseases of heart--------------------------390-398,402,404,410-429	227	1.8
7	Meningitis--320	220	1.8
8	Cerebrovascular diseases------------------------------------430-438	90	0.7
8	Meningococcal infections------------------------------------036	90	0.7
10	Enteritis and other diarrheal diseases----------------------008,009	82	0.7
	1-4 years, male		
	All causes--	4,915	78.2
1	Accidents--E800-E949	2,087	33.2
2	Congenital anomalies--740-759	550	8.7
3	Malignant neoplasms, including neoplasms of lymphatic and hematopoietic tissues--------------------------------------140-209	352	5.6
4	Influenza and pneumonia-------------------------470-474,480-486	250	4.0
5	Homicide--E960-E978	154	2.4
6	Meningitis--320	152	2.4
7	Diseases of heart--------------------------390-398,402,404,410-429	133	2.1
8	Meningococcal infections------------------------------------036	52	0.8
9	Cerebrovascular diseases------------------------------------430-438	50	0.8
10	Enteritis and other diarrheal diseases----------------------008,009	41	0.7
	1-4 years, female		
	All causes--	3,691	61.3
1	Accidents--E800-E949	1,352	22.4
2	Congenital anomalies--740-759	564	9.4
3	Malignant neoplasms, including neoplasms of lymphatic and hematopoietic tissues--------------------------------------140-209	304	5.0
4	Influenza and pneumonia-------------------------470-474,480-486	230	3.8
5	Homicide--E960-E978	152	2.5
6	Diseases of heart--------------------------390-398,402,404,410-429	94	1.6
7	Meningitis--320	68	1.1
8	Enteritis and other diarrheal diseases----------------------008,009	41	0.7
9	Cerebrovascular diseases------------------------------------430-438	40	0.7
10	Meningococcal infections------------------------------------036	38	0.6
10	Septicemia--038	38	0.6

Table 28. Deaths and death rates for the 10 leading causes of death in specified age and sex groups: 1976—Con.

Rank	Age, sex, cause of death, and category numbers of the Eighth Revision International Classification of Diseases, Adapted, 1965	Number	Rate per 100,000 population in specified group
	5-14 years, both sexes		
	All causes--	12,901	34.7
1	Accidents---E800-E949	6,308	17.0
2	Malignant neoplasms, including neoplasms of lymphatic and hematopoietic tissues-------------------------------------140-209	1,849	5.0
3	Congenital anomalies---740-759	745	2.0
4	Homicide--E960-E978	392	1.1
5	Influenza and pneumonia----------------------------470-474,480-486	362	1.0
6	Diseases of heart-------------------------390-398,402,404,410-429	332	0.9
7	Cerebrovascular diseases-----------------------------------430-438	206	0.6
8	Suicide---E950-E959	163	0.4
9	Benign neoplasms and neoplasms of unspecified nature--------210-239	112	0.3
10	Anemias---280-285	98	0.3
	5-14 years, male		
	All causes--	8,068	42.6
1	Accidents---E800-E949	4,343	22.9
2	Malignant neoplasms, including neoplasms of lymphatic and hematopoietic tissues-------------------------------------140-209	1,105	5.8
3	Congenital anomalies---740-759	367	1.9
4	Homicide--E960-E978	240	1.3
5	Influenza and pneumonia----------------------------470-474,480-486	177	0.9
6	Diseases of heart-------------------------390-398,402,404,410-429	174	0.9
7	Suicide---E950-E959	126	0.7
8	Cerebrovascular diseases-----------------------------------430-438	118	0.6
9	Benign neoplasms and neoplasms of unspecified nature--------210-239	72	0.4
10	Anemias---280-285	50	0.3
	5-14 years, female		
	All causes--	4,833	26.5
1	Accidents---E800-E949	1,965	10.8
2	Malignant neoplasms, including neoplasms of lymphatic and hematopoietic tissues-------------------------------------140-209	744	4.1
3	Congenital anomalies---740-759	378	2.1
4	Influenza and pneumonia----------------------------470-474,480,486	185	1.0
5	Diseases of heart-------------------------390-398,402,404,410-429	158	0.9
6	Homicide--E960-E978	152	0.8
7	Cerebrovascular diseases-----------------------------------430-438	88	0.5
8	Anemias---280-285	48	0.3
9	Meningitis--320	43	0.2
10	Benign neoplasms and neoplasms of unspecified nature--------210-239	40	0.2

Table 28. Deaths and death rates for the 10 leading causes of death in specified age and sex groups: 1976—Con.

Rank	Age, sex, cause of death, and category numbers of the Eighth Revision International Classification of Diseases, Adapted, 1965	Number	Rate per 100,000 population in specified group
	15-24 years, both sexes		
	All causes---	46,081	113.5
1	Accidents--E800-E949	24,316	59.9
2	Homicide---E960-E978	5,038	12.4
3	Suicide--E950-E959	4,747	11.7
4	Malignant neoplasms, including neoplasms of lymphatic and hematopoietic tissues---140-209	2,659	6.5
5	Diseases of heart---------------------------390-398,402,404,410-429	1,072	2.6
6	Influenza and pneumonia--------------------------------470-474,480-486	611	1.5
7	Congenital anomalies---740-759	568	1.4
8	Cerebrovascular diseases---------------------------------------430-438	506	1.2
9	Diabetes mellitus---250	159	0.4
10	Anemias--280-285	138	0.3
	15-24 years, male		
	All causes---	34,253	167.7
1	Accidents--E800-E949	19,214	94.1
2	Homicide---E960-E978	3,907	19.1
3	Suicide--E950-E959	3,786	18.5
4	Malignant neoplasms, including neoplasms of lymphatic and hematopoietic tissues---140-209	1,628	8.0
5	Diseases of heart---------------------------390-398,402,404,410-429	690	3.4
6	Influenza and pneumonia--------------------------------470-474,480-486	336	1.6
7	Congenital anomalies---740-759	329	1.6
8	Cerebrovascular diseases---------------------------------------430-438	281	1.4
9	Anemias--280-285	86	0.4
10	Nephritis and nephrosis--580-584	76	0.4
	15-24 years, female		
	All causes---	11,828	58.6
1	Accidents--E800-E949	5,102	25.3
2	Homicide---E960-E978	1,131	5.6
3	Malignant neoplasms, including neoplasms of lymphatic and hematopoietic tissues---140-209	1,031	5.1
4	Suicide--E950-E959	961	4.8
5	Diseases of heart---------------------------390-398,402,404,410-429	382	1.9
6	Influenza and pneumonia--------------------------------470-474,480-486	275	1.4
7	Congenital anomalies---740-759	239	1.2
8	Cerebrovascular diseases---------------------------------------430-438	225	1.1
9	Complications of pregnancy, childbirth, and the puerperium---630-678	137	0.7
10	Diabetes mellitus---250	85	0.4

Table 28. Deaths and death rates for the 10 leading causes of death in specified age and sex groups: 1976—Con.

Rank	Age, sex, cause of death, and category numbers of the Eighth Revision International Classification of Diseases, Adapted, 1965	Number	Rate per 100,000 population in specified group
	25-44 years, both sexes		
	All causes---	101,898	185.6
1	Accidents---E800-E949	22,399	40.8
2	Malignant neoplasms, including neoplasms of lymphatic and hematopoietic tissues------------------------------------140-209	16,485	30.0
3	Diseases of heart---------------------------390-398,402,404,410-429	14,393	26.2
4	Suicide---E950-E959	8,823	16.1
5	Homicide--E960-E978	8,554	15.6
6	Cirrhosis of liver---571	5,058	9.2
7	Cerebrovascular diseases--------------------------------430-438	3,737	6.8
8	Influenza and pneumonia--------------------------470-474,480-486	2,027	3.7
9	Diabetes mellitus---250	1,477	2.7
10	Congenital anomalies------------------------------------740-759	740	1.3
	25-44 years, male		
	All causes---	67,322	249.6
1	Accidents---E800-E949	17,730	65.7
2	Diseases of heart---------------------------390-398,402,404,410-429	10,865	40.3
3	Malignant neoplasms, including neoplasms of lymphatic and hematopoietic tissues------------------------------------140-209	7,420	27.5
4	Homicide--E960-E978	6,930	25.7
5	Suicide---E950-E959	6,273	23.3
6	Cirrhosis of liver---571	3,356	12.4
7	Cerebrovascular diseases--------------------------------430-438	1,826	6.8
8	Influenza and pneumonia--------------------------470-474,480-486	1,191	4.4
9	Diabetes mellitus---250	826	3.1
10	Congenital anomalies------------------------------------740-759	400	1.5
	25-44 years, female		
	All causes---	34,576	123.8
1	Malignant neoplasms, including neoplasms of lymphatic and hematopoietic tissues------------------------------------140-209	9,065	32.5
2	Accidents---E800-E949	4,669	16.7
3	Diseases of heart---------------------------390-398,402,404,410-429	3,528	12.6
4	Suicide---E950-E959	2,550	9.1
5	Cerebrovascular diseases--------------------------------430-438	1,911	6.8
6	Cirrhosis of liver---571	1,702	6.1
7	Homicide--E960-E978	1,624	5.8
8	Influenza and pneumonia--------------------------470-474,480-486	836	3.0
9	Diabetes mellitus---250	651	2.3
10	Congenital anomalies------------------------------------740-759	340	1.2

Table 28. Deaths and death rates for the 10 leading causes of death in specified age and sex groups: 1976—Con.

Rank	Age, sex, cause of death, and category numbers of the Eighth Revision International Classification of Diseases, Adapted, 1965	Number	Rate per 100,000 population in specified group
	45-64 years, both sexes		
	All causes--	446,096	1,020.8
1	Diseases of heart----------------------------390-398,402,404,410-429	158,069	361.7
2	Malignant neoplasms, including neoplasms of lymphatic and hematopoietic tissues--140-209	130,993	299.8
3	Cerebrovascular diseases-------------------------------------430-438	24,630	56.4
4	Accidents--E800-E949	19,000	43.5
5	Cirrhosis of liver---571	17,821	40.8
6	Suicide--E950-E959	8,546	19.6
7	Influenza and pneumonia--------------------------470-474,480-486	8,010	18.3
8	Diabetes mellitus--250	8,006	18.3
9	Bronchitis, emphysema, and asthma---------------------------490-493	6,040	13.8
10	Homicide---E960-E978	3,837	8.8
	45-64 years, male		
	All causes--	285,019	1,362.6
1	Diseases of heart----------------------------390-398,402,404,410-429	116,062	554.9
2	Malignant neoplasms, including neoplasms of lymphatic and hematopoietic tissues--140-209	70,847	338.7
3	Accidents--E800-E949	13,595	65.0
4	Cerebrovascular diseases-------------------------------------430-438	13,196	63.1
5	Cirrhosis of liver---571	11,900	56.9
6	Suicide--E950-E959	5,816	27.8
7	Influenza and pneumonia--------------------------470-474,480-486	5,159	24.7
8	Bronchitis, emphysema, and asthma---------------------------490-493	4,089	19.5
9	Diabetes mellitus--250	3,824	18.3
10	Homicide---E960-E978	3,022	14.4
	45-64 years, female		
	All causes--	161,077	707.0
1	Malignant neoplasms, including neoplasms of lymphatic and hematopoietic tissues--140-209	60,146	264.0
2	Diseases of heart----------------------------390-398,402,404,410-429	42,007	184.4
3	Cerebrovascular diseases-------------------------------------430-438	11,434	50.2
4	Cirrhosis of liver---571	5,921	26.0
5	Accidents--E800-E949	5,405	23.7
6	Diabetes mellitus--250	4,182	18.4
7	Influenza and pneumonia--------------------------470-474,480-486	2,851	12.5
8	Suicide--E950-E959	2,730	12.0
9	Bronchitis, emphysema, and asthma---------------------------490-493	1,951	8.6
10	Nephritis and nephrosis-------------------------------------580-584	893	3.9

Table 28. Deaths and death rates for the 10 leading causes of death in specified age and sex groups: 1976—Con.

Rank	Age, sex, cause of death, and category numbers of the Eighth Revision International Classification of Diseases, Adapted, 1965	Number	Rate per 100,000 population in specified group
	65 years and over, both sexes		
	All causes---	1,245,118	5,428.9
1	Diseases of heart----------------------------390-398,402,404,410-429	548,956	2,393.5
2	Malignant neoplasms, including neoplasms of lymphatic and		
	hematopoietic tissues--140-209	224,543	979.0
3	Cerebrovascular diseases-------------------------------------430-438	159,304	694.6
4	Influenza and pneumonia----------------------------470-474,480-486	48,405	211.1
5	Arteriosclerosis---440	28,032	122.2
6	Diabetes mellitus---250	24,797	108.1
7	Accidents--E800-E949	23,961	104.5
8	Bronchitis, emphysema, and asthma---------------------------490-493	17,623	76.8
9	Cirrhosis of liver---571	8,378	36.5
10	Nephritis and nephrosis---------------------------------------580-584	5,732	25.0
	65 years and over, male		
	All causes---	624,778	6,672.1
1	Diseases of heart----------------------------390-398,402,404,410-429	272,205	2,906.9
2	Malignant neoplasms, including neoplasms of lymphatic and		
	hematopoietic tissues--140-209	123,983	1,324.0
3	Cerebrovascular diseases-------------------------------------430-438	65,052	694.7
4	Influenza and pneumonia----------------------------470-474,480-486	24,307	259.6
5	Bronchitis, emphysema, and asthma---------------------------490-493	13,315	142.2
6	Accidents--E800-E949	12,527	133.8
7	Arteriosclerosis---440	10,963	117.1
8	Diabetes mellitus---250	9,273	99.0
9	Cirrhosis of liver---571	5,297	56.6
10	Suicide--E950-E959	3,489	37.3
	65 years and over, female		
	All causes---	620,340	4,571.1
1	Diseases of heart----------------------------390-398,402,404,410-429	276,751	2,039.3
2	Malignant neoplasms, including neoplasms of lymphatic and		
	hematopoietic tissues--140-209	100,560	741.0
3	Cerebrovascular diseases-------------------------------------430-438	94,252	694.5
4	Influenza and pneumonia----------------------------470-474,480-486	24,098	177.6
5	Arteriosclerosis---440	17,069	125.8
6	Diabetes mellitus---250	15,524	114.4
7	Accidents--E800-E949	11,434	84.3
8	Bronchitis, emphysema, and asthma---------------------------490-493	4,308	31.7
9	Cirrhosis of liver---571	3,081	22.7
10	Nephritis and nephrosis---------------------------------------580-584	2,763	20.4

Selected Causes

Table 29. Age-adjusted death rates for 69 selected causes of death: 1970 and 1976

[Refers only to resident deaths occurring within the United States. Excludes fetal deaths. Based on age-specific death rates per 100,000 estimated midyear population in specified group. Computed by the direct method, using as the standard population the age distribution of the total population of the United States as enumerated in 1940]

Cause of death and category numbers of the Eighth Revision International Classification of Diseases, Adapted, 1965	1976	1970
All causes--	627.5	714.3
Bacillary dysentery and amebiasis---------------------------------------004,006	0.0	0.0
Enteritis and other diarrheal diseases----------------------------------008,009	0.7	1.0
Tuberculosis, all forms---010-019	1.1	2.2
Tuberculosis of respiratory system-------------------------------------010-012	0.9	1.7
Tuberculosis, other forms--013-019	0.3	0.5
Whooping cough--033	0.0	0.0
Streptococcal sore throat and scarlet fever-------------------------------034	0.0	0.0
Meningococcal infections--036	0.2	0.3
Septicemia--038	2.3	1.4
Acute poliomyelitis---040-043	0.0	0.0
Measles---055	0.0	0.0
Syphilis and its sequelae---090-097	0.1	0.2
Other infective and parasitic diseases----------------------Remainder of 000-136	1.7	1.8
Malignant neoplasms, including neoplasms of lymphatic and hematopoietic tissues--140-209	132.3	129.9
Malignant neoplasms of buccal cavity and pharynx-----------------------140-149	3.0	3.1
Malignant neoplasms of digestive organs and peritoneum-----------------150-159	33.6	35.2
Malignant neoplasms of respiratory system-----------------------------160-163	33.5	28.4
Malignant neoplasm of breast--174	12.6	12.6
Malignant neoplasms of genital organs--------------------------------180-187	14.7	15.6
Malignant neoplasms of urinary organs------------------------------188,189	5.5	5.7
Malignant neoplasms of all other and unspecified sites----------170-173,190-199	16.8	15.9
Leukemia--204-207	5.4	5.8
Other neoplasms of lymphatic and hematopoietic tissues----------200-203,208,209	7.3	7.7
Benign neoplasms and neoplasms of unspecified nature---------------------210-239	1.7	2.0
Diabetes mellitus---250	11.1	14.1
Avitaminoses and other nutritional deficiencies----------------------260-269	0.7	0.8
Anemias--280-285	1.0	1.3
Meningitis--320	0.7	0.8
Major cardiovascular diseases--390-448	284.4	340.1
Diseases of heart-----------------------------------390-398,402,404,410-429	216.7	253.6
Active rheumatic fever and chronic rheumatic heart disease-------------390-398	4.7	6.3
Hypertensive heart disease---402	2.0	2.9
Hypertensive heart and renal disease-----------------------------------404	1.0	2.0
Ischemic heart disease---410-413	191.6	228.1
Acute myocardial infarction--410	102.9	130.4
Other acute and subacute forms of ischemic heart disease-----------411	1.3	1.6
Chronic ischemic heart disease------------------------------------412	87.3	96.0
Angina pectoris---413	0.1	0.1
Chronic disease of endocardium and other myocardial insufficiency--424,428	1.3	2.3
All other forms of heart disease-------------------420-423,425-427,429	16.1	12.0
Hypertension---400,401,403	1.8	2.9
Cerebrovascular diseases--430-438	51.4	66.3
Cerebral hemorrhage---431	8.0	14.6
Cerebral thrombosis---433	11.4	17.3
Cerebral embolism---434	0.2	0.3
All other cerebrovascular diseases----------------------430,432,435-438	31.8	34.1
Arteriosclerosis--440	6.4	8.4
Other diseases of arteries, arterioles, and capillaries-------------441-448	8.0	8.8
Acute bronchitis and bronchiolitis-------------------------------------466	0.3	0.5
Influenza and pneumonia--470-474,480-486	17.4	22.1
Influenza---470-474	1.9	1.3
Pneumonia---480-486	15.5	20.8

Table 29. Age-adjusted death rates for 69 selected causes of death: 1970 and 1976—Con.

[Refers only to resident deaths occurring within the United States. Excludes fetal deaths. Based on age-specific death rates per 100,000 estimated midyear population in specified group. Computed by the direct method, using as the standard population the age distribution of the total population of the United States as enumerated in 1940]

Cause of death and category numbers of the Eighth Revision International Classification of Diseases, Adapted, 1965	1976	1970
Bronchitis, emphysema, and asthma---490-493	7.9	11.6
Chronic and unqualified bronchitis---490,491	1.5	2.1
Emphysema---492	5.7	8.4
Asthma---493	0.8	1.0
Peptic ulcer---531-533	2.1	3.2
Appendicitis---540-543	0.3	0.6
Hernia and intestinal obstruction---550-553,560	1.8	2.6
Cirrhosis of liver---571	13.6	14.7
Cholelithiasis, cholecystitis and cholangitis---574,575	0.8	1.3
Nephritis and nephrosis---580-584	2.8	3.5
Acute nephritis and nephrotic syndrome---580,581	0.5	0.6
Chronic and unqualified nephritis and renal sclerosis---582-584	2.3	3.0
Infections of kidney---590	1.1	2.8
Hyperplasia of prostate---600	0.3	0.6
Complications of pregnancy, childbirth, and the puerperium---630-678	0.2	0.5
Abortions---640-645	0.0	0.1
Other complications of pregnancy, childbirth, and the puerperium---630-639,650-678	0.2	0.4
Congenital anomalies---740-759	6.4	7.6
Certain causes of mortality in early infancy---760-769.2,769.4-772,774-778	12.6	19.0
Birth injury, difficult labor, and other anoxic and hypoxic conditions---764-768,772,776	6.8	10.0
Other causes of mortality in early infancy---Remainder of 760-778	5.8	9.0
Symptoms and ill-defined conditions---780-796	11.6	10.4
All other diseases---Residual	43.1	40.2
Accidents---E800-E949	43.2	53.7
Motor vehicle accidents---E810-E823	21.5	27.4
All other accidents---E800-E807,E825-E949	21.7	26.3
Suicide---E950-E959	12.3	11.8
Homicide---E960-E978	9.5	9.1
Other external causes---E980-E999	2.2	2.8

Table 30. Death rates for Diseases of heart by color and sex: Selected years, 1950-76

[Rates per 100,000 population in specified group]

Year	Total			White			All other		
	Both sexes	Male	Fe-male	Both sexes	Male	Fe-male	Both sexes	Male	Fe-male
1976[1]	337.2	383.5	293.4	351.3	399.4	305.5	244.8	276.5	215.9
1975[1]	336.2	385.2	289.7	350.0	401.1	301.3	244.4	277.1	214.7
1974[1]	349.2	399.7	301.2	362.7	415.5	312.3	258.0	291.0	227.9
1973[1]	360.8	415.2	309.1	373.9	430.9	319.4	271.3	305.9	239.7
1972[1,2]	363.0	418.5	310.3	376.2	434.1	321.0	271.5	308.4	237.6
1971[1]	360.5	417.9	306.0	373.6	433.9	316.1	268.9	303.9	236.7
1970[1]	362.0	422.5	304.5	374.5	438.3	313.8	274.2	310.2	241.0
1969[a]	367.1	430.5	307.0	379.1	445.7	315.7	281.2	319.6	246.0
1968[a]	373.5	438.4	311.8	384.7	453.2	319.4	292.4	330.0	257.8
1967[a]	365.3	431.8	302.0	377.6	447.9	310.4	275.7	312.6	241.6
1966[a]	371.7	439.2	307.1	383.2	454.4	314.8	287.4	325.6	252.0
1965[a]	368.0	435.3	303.2	379.5	450.8	310.7	282.4	318.4	248.6
1960	369.0	439.5	300.6	379.6	454.6	306.5	287.1	320.5	255.5
1955	356.5	425.8	289.0	364.9	438.5	293.0	287.2	319.4	256.8
1950	356.8	424.7	289.7	362.0	434.2	290.5	311.8	432.0	283.0

[1] Excludes deaths of nonresidents of the United States.
[2] Based on a 50-percent sample of deaths.
[a] Revised.

Table 31. Deaths and death rates for Diseases of heart by age and sex: 1976

Age	Number			Rate per 100,000 population in specified group		
	Both sexes	Male	Female	Both sexes	Male	Female
All ages	723,878	400,601	323,277	337.2	383.5	293.4
Under 1 year	700	404	296	23.1	26.1	20.1
1-4 years	227	133	94	1.8	2.1	1.6
5-14 years	332	174	158	0.9	0.9	0.9
15-24 years	1,072	690	382	2.6	3.4	1.9
25-34 years	2,706	1,884	822	8.5	12.0	5.1
35-44 years	11,687	8,981	2,706	50.8	80.1	22.9
45-54 years	47,230	36,311	10,919	199.8	317.7	89.5
55-64 years	110,839	79,751	31,088	552.4	840.6	293.9
65-74 years	182,667	113,941	68,726	1,286.9	1,847.6	856.2
75-84 years	221,113	106,215	114,898	3,263.7	4,136.1	2,731.1
85 years and over	145,176	52,049	93,127	7,384.3	8,274.9	6,965.4
Age not stated	129	68	61	...	...	...

Table 32. Death rates for Malignant neoplasms, including neoplasms of lymphatic and hematopoietic tissues by color and sex: Selected years, 1950-76

[Rates per 100,000 population in specified group]

Year	Total			White			All other		
	Both sexes	Male	Female	Both sexes	Male	Female	Both sexes	Male	Female
1976[1]	175.8	196.6	156.0	180.2	199.2	162.0	147.1	179.2	117.8
1975[1]	171.7	192.3	152.1	175.8	194.8	157.7	144.0	175.3	115.5
1974[1]	170.5	191.1	151.0	174.4	193.7	156.1	144.1	173.5	117.2
1973[1]	167.3	187.1	148.4	170.9	189.6	153.0	142.8	170.1	117.9
1972 [1,2]	166.0	185.7	147.2	170.0	188.7	152.2	138.2	165.2	113.4
1971[1]	163.6	183.1	145.1	167.4	186.1	149.5	137.4	161.8	115.0
1970[1]	162.8	182.1	144.4	166.8	185.1	149.4	134.4	161.0	110.0
1969[a]	160.4	179.7	142.1	163.9	182.3	146.4	135.4	160.8	112.0
1968[a]	159.8	178.8	141.6	163.2	181.5	145.7	135.1	159.2	112.9
1967[a]	157.5	175.6	140.2	161.0	178.5	144.3	131.7	154.3	110.9
1966[a]	155.3	172.5	138.8	158.7	175.4	142.7	130.3	151.0	111.0
1965[a]	153.8	170.2	138.0	157.5	173.7	141.9	126.1	144.3	109.2
1960	149.2	162.5	136.4	152.8	166.1	139.8	121.6	134.1	109.8
1955	146.5	155.8	137.4	150.4	160.0	141.0	114.0	119.9	108.4
1950	139.8	142.9	136.8	143.5	147.2	139.9	108.1	106.1	110.1

[1]Excludes deaths of nonresidents of the United States.
[2]Based on a 50-percent sample of deaths.
[a]Revised.

Table 33. Deaths and death rates for Malignant neoplasms, including neoplasms of lymphatic and hematopoietic tissues by age and sex: 1976

Age	Number			Rate per 100,000 population in specified group		
	Both sexes	Male	Female	Both sexes	Male	Female
All ages	377,312	205,406	171,906	175.8	196.6	156.0
Under 1 year	98	52	46	3.2	3.4	3.1
1-4 years	656	352	304	5.3	5.6	5.0
5-14 years	1,849	1,105	744	5.0	5.8	4.1
15-24 years	2,659	1,628	1,031	6.5	8.0	5.1
25-34 years	4,629	2,203	2,426	14.5	14.0	15.0
35-44 years	11,856	5,217	6,639	51.5	46.6	56.2
45-54 years	43,025	21,480	21,545	182.0	187.9	176.5
55-64 years	87,968	49,367	38,601	438.4	520.4	364.9
65-74 years	111,611	65,375	46,236	786.3	1,060.1	576.0
75-84 years	84,592	45,764	38,828	1,248.6	1,782.1	922.9
85 years and over	28,340	12,844	15,496	1,441.5	2,042.0	1,159.0
Age not stated	29	19	10	...	...	...

Table 34. Death rates for Cerebrovascular diseases by color and sex: Selected years, 1950-76

[Rates per 100,000 population in specified group]

Year	Total			White			All other		
	Both sexes	Male	Female	Both sexes	Male	Female	Both sexes	Male	Female
1976[1] ----------------------	87.9	77.1	98.0	88.9	76.8	100.5	80.9	79.3	82.3
1975[1] ----------------------	91.1	81.3	100.4	92.2	81.1	102.8	83.7	82.4	84.9
1974[1] ----------------------	98.1	87.8	107.9	99.2	87.6	110.3	90.9	89.4	92.3
1973[1] ----------------------	102.1	91.8	111.9	102.7	91.2	113.7	98.1	96.1	99.9
1972[1,2] ----------------------	102.5	94.0	110.5	103.0	93.6	112.0	98.7	96.6	100.6
1971[1] ----------------------	101.4	93.8	108.6	101.7	93.2	109.9	99.0	98.0	99.9
1970[1] ----------------------	101.9	94.5	109.0	101.9	93.5	109.8	102.6	101.6	103.5
1969[a] ----------------------	102.9	96.2	109.3	102.4	94.7	109.6	106.5	106.4	106.6
1968[a] ----------------------	106.0	99.6	112.1	105.1	97.8	112.1	112.4	112.5	112.3
1967[a] ----------------------	102.4	96.6	107.9	101.8	95.4	108.0	106.4	105.7	107.0
1966[a] ----------------------	104.7	98.9	110.3	103.7	97.1	110.0	112.3	112.1	112.5
1965[a] ----------------------	103.9	98.6	109.0	102.4	96.5	108.0	114.9	114.2	115.6
1960-------------------------	108.0	104.5	111.4	106.4	102.7	110.1	119.7	118.2	121.2
1955-------------------------	106.0	104.0	107.9	104.3	102.3	106.2	119.9	118.0	121.8
1950-------------------------	104.0	102.5	105.6	101.9	100.5	103.3	122.3	119.5	124.9

[1]Excludes deaths of nonresidents of the United States.
[2]Based on a 50-percent sample of deaths.
[a]Revised.

Table 35. Death rates for Arteriosclerosis by color and sex: Selected years, 1950-76

[Rates per 100,000 population in specified group]

Year	Total			White			All other		
	Both sexes	Male	Female	Both sexes	Male	Female	Both sexes	Male	Female
1976[1] ----------------------	13.7	11.3	15.9	14.7	12.0	17.2	7.3	6.8	7.8
1975[1] ----------------------	13.6	11.4	15.6	14.5	12.0	16.9	7.4	7.4	7.5
1974[1] ----------------------	15.3	12.9	17.5	16.2	13.5	18.9	8.5	8.3	8.7
1973[1] ----------------------	15.5	13.1	17.9	16.5	13.8	19.1	8.9	8.5	9.2
1972[1,2] ----------------------	15.6	13.5	17.6	16.5	14.1	18.8	9.3	9.4	9.3
1971[1] ----------------------	15.3	13.3	17.2	16.2	14.0	18.4	8.6	8.2	9.0
1970[1] ----------------------	15.6	13.9	17.2	16.6	14.6	18.4	8.9	8.9	8.9
1969[a] ----------------------	16.4	14.6	18.1	17.4	15.3	19.3	9.7	9.8	9.5
1968[a] ----------------------	16.8	15.1	18.5	17.8	15.7	19.7	10.2	10.3	10.0
1967[a] ----------------------	19.0	17.2	20.7	20.1	18.0	22.1	10.9	11.2	10.7
1966[a] ----------------------	19.9	18.3	21.5	20.9	19.1	22.8	12.2	12.4	12.0
1965[a] ----------------------	19.7	18.2	21.1	20.7	19.0	22.3	12.2	12.5	11.9
1960-------------------------	20.0	19.3	20.7	20.9	20.0	21.8	13.0	14.0	12.0
1955-------------------------	19.8	19.9	19.7	20.6	20.5	20.7	12.9	14.2	11.7
1950-------------------------	20.4	20.9	19.8	21.3	21.7	20.9	12.8	14.4	11.3

[1]Excludes deaths of nonresidents of the United States.
[2]Based on a 50-percent sample of deaths.
[a]Revised.

Table 36. Death rates for Bronchitis, emphysema, and asthma by color and sex:. Selected years, 1950-76

[Rates per 100,000 population in specified group]

Year	Total			White			All other		
	Both sexes	Male	Female	Both sexes	Male	Female	Both sexes	Male	Female
1976[1]	11.4	17.0	6.0	12.3	18.3	6.5	5.5	8.2	3.0
1975[1]	12.0	18.3	6.0	12.9	19.7	6.4	5.9	8.6	3.3
1974[1]	12.7	19.6	6.2	13.7	21.1	6.7	6.0	9.2	3.1
1973[1]	14.2	22.2	6.5	15.2	23.9	6.9	7.0	10.7	3.6
1972[1,2]	14.8	23.3	6.7	15.8	25.0	7.1	7.5	11.3	4.1
1971[1]	14.7	23.4	6.4	15.7	25.0	6.8	7.8	11.5	4.3
1970[1]	15.2	24.4	6.4	16.2	26.1	6.7	8.4	12.5	4.6
1969[a]	15.5	25.2	6.3	16.4	26.8	6.5	8.8	13.3	4.7
1968[a]	16.6	27.0	6.7	17.5	28.7	6.9	9.8	14.8	5.2
1967[a]	15.4	25.2	6.0	16.2	26.8	6.2	9.0	13.4	4.9
1966[a]	15.2	25.0	5.8	16.1	26.6	6.0	8.7	13.2	4.5
1965[a]	14.4	23.7	5.6	15.2	25.1	5.7	8.7	13.1	4.5
1960	9.9	15.8	4.3	10.3	16.5	4.2	7.4	10.0	4.9
1955	7.0	10.5	3.7	7.3	10.9	3.7	5.3	7.0	3.6
1950	5.0	6.6	3.3	5.0	6.8	3.3	4.5	5.4	3.6

[1]Excludes deaths of nonresidents of the United States.
[2]Based on a 50-percent sample of deaths.
[a]Revised.

Table 37. Deaths and death rates for Bronchitis, emphysema, and asthma by age and sex: 1976

Age	Number			Rate per 100,000 population in specified group		
	Both sexes	Male	Female	Both sexes	Male	Female
All ages	24,410	17,784	6,626	11.4	17.0	6.0
Under 1 year	71	44	27	2.3	2.8	1.8
1-4 years	61	34	27	0.5	0.5	0.4
5-14 years	58	30	28	0.2	0.2	0.2
15-24 years	96	52	44	0.2	0.3	0.2
25-34 years	149	72	77	0.5	0.5	0.5
35-44 years	310	147	163	1.3	1.3	1.4
45-54 years	1,423	855	568	6.0	7.5	4.7
55-64 years	4,617	3,234	1,383	23.0	34.1	13.1
65-74 years	8,618	6,646	1,972	60.7	107.8	24.6
75-84 years	6,872	5,228	1,644	101.4	203.6	39.1
85 years and over	2,133	1,441	692	108.5	229.1	51.8
Age not stated	2	1	1	...	...	...

Table 38. Death rates for Accidents by color and sex: Selected years, 1950-76

[Rates per 100,000 population in specified group]

Year	Total			White			All other		
	Both sexes	Male	Female	Both sexes	Male	Female	Both sexes	Male	Female
1976[1]-------------------	46.9	67.3	27.7	46.3	65.6	27.9	51.3	78.7	26.3
1975[1]-------------------	48.4	69.8	28.0	47.4	67.7	28.0	54.7	84.1	28.0
1974[1]-------------------	49.5	71.1	29.0	48.5	69.1	28.9	56.0	85.3	29.3
1973[1]-------------------	55.2	78.7	32.8	53.8	75.9	32.7	64.6	98.5	33.6
1972[1,2]-----------------	55.4	78.6	33.4	54.0	75.6	33.4	65.4	99.8	33.8
1971[1]-------------------	55.0	77.9	33.3	53.3	74.6	33.0	67.0	101.2	35.7
1970[1]-------------------	56.4	80.6	33.4	54.6	77.2	33.1	68.8	105.0	35.5
1969[a]-------------------	57.8	82.4	34.5	56.0	79.0	34.1	70.5	106.9	37.2
1968[a]-------------------	57.6	81.8	34.7	55.7	78.0	34.3	71.6	109.2	37.0
1967[a]-------------------	57.3	80.9	34.9	55.8	77.8	34.6	68.6	103.2	36.6
1966[a]-------------------	58.1	81.5	35.6	56.3	78.3	35.1	71.4	105.3	39.9
1965[a]-------------------	55.8	78.1	34.4	54.3	75.3	34.0	67.2	99.3	37.2
1960---------------------	52.3	72.8	32.4	50.5	70.0	31.5	66.1	95.0	38.7
1955---------------------	56.9	79.8	34.5	55.3	77.3	33.8	70.0	100.9	40.7
1950---------------------	60.6	84.7	36.7	59.3	82.5	36.3	71.2	103.9	39.9

[1]Excludes deaths of nonresidents of the United States.
[2]Based on a 50-percent sample of deaths.
[a]Revised.

Table 39. Deaths and death rates for Motor vehicle accidents and All other accidents in order of frequency: 1976

Cause of death and category numbers of the Eighth Revision International Classification of Diseases, Adapted, 1965	Number	Rate[1]
All accidents--E800-E949	100,761	46.9
Motor vehicle accidents---E810-E823	47,038	21.9
All other accidents-----------------------------------E800-E807,E825-E949	53,723	25.0
Accidental falls--E880-E887	14,136	6.6
Accidents caused by fires and flames------------------------------E890-E899	6,338	3.0
Accidental drowning and submersion-------------------------------------E910	5,645	2.6
Accidental poisoning by solid and liquid substances---------------E850-E869	4,161	1.9
Inhalation and ingestion of food or other object causing obstruction or suffocation---------------------------------E911,E912	3,033	1.4
Surgical and medical complications and misadventures---------------E930-E936	3,009	1.4
Accident caused by firearm missile------------------------------------E922	2,059	1.0
Striking against or struck accidentally by objects, including falling objects--E916,E917	1,875	0.9
Accidental poisoning by gases and vapors--------------------------E870-E877	1,569	0.7
Air and space transport accidents--------------------------------E840-E845	1,445	0.7
Water transport accidents--E830-E838	1,371	0.6
Accidents due to natural and environmental factors----------------E900-E909	1,299	0.6
Accidents caused by electric current----------------------------------E925	1,041	0.5
Accidental mechanical suffocation-------------------------------------E913	911	0.4
Late effects of accidental injuries------------------------------E940-E949	778	0.4
Machinery accidents not elsewhere classifiable------------------------E928	768	0.4
Railway accidents--E800-E807	552	0.3
Caught accidentally in or between objects-----------------------------E918	471	0.2
Accident caused by explosive material---------------------------------E923	442	0.2
Other road vehicle accidents-------------------------------------E825-E827	238	0.1
Accident caused by hot substance, corrosive liquid, and steam---------E924	210	0.1
Vehicle accidents not elsewhere classifiable-------------------------E927	170	0.1
Accident caused by cutting or piercing instrument--------------------E920	135	0.1
Residual---------------------------------E914,E915,E919,E921,E926,E929	2,067	1.0

[1]Rate per 100,000 population.

Table 40. Death rates for Suicide by color and sex: Selected years, 1950-76

[Rates per 100,000 population in specified group]

Year	Total			White			All other		
	Both sexes	Male	Female	Both sexes	Male	Female	Both sexes	Male	Female
1976[1]	12.5	18.7	6.7	13.3	19.8	7.2	7.0	11.0	3.2
1975[1]	12.7	18.9	6.8	13.6	20.1	7.4	6.8	10.6	3.3
1974[1]	12.1	18.1	6.5	13.0	19.2	7.1	6.5	10.2	3.0
1973[1]	12.0	17.7	6.5	12.8	18.8	7.0	6.4	10.0	3.0
1972[1,2]	12.0	17.5	6.8	12.8	18.5	7.3	6.6	10.3	3.3
1971[1]	11.7	16.8	6.8	12.5	17.9	7.3	5.9	8.6	3.4
1970[1]	11.6	16.8	6.6	12.4	18.0	7.1	5.6	8.5	2.9
1969[a]	11.1	16.2	6.3	11.9	17.3	6.8	5.4	8.2	2.7
1968[a]	10.7	15.8	5.9	11.5	17.0	6.4	4.8	7.4	2.4
1967[a]	10.8	15.8	6.1	11.6	16.9	6.5	5.1	7.7	2.7
1966[a]	10.9	16.1	5.9	11.7	17.2	6.3	5.0	7.9	2.4
1965[a]	11.1	16.3	6.1	11.9	17.5	6.6	5.1	7.8	2.5
1960	10.6	16.5	4.9	11.4	17.6	5.3	4.5	7.2	2.0
1955	10.2	16.0	4.6	11.0	17.2	4.9	3.8	6.1	1.5
1950	11.4	17.8	5.1	12.2	19.0	5.5	4.3	7.0	1.7

[1]Excludes deaths of nonresidents of the United States.
[2]Based on a 50-percent sample of deaths.
[a]Revised.

Table 41. Deaths and death rates for Suicide by age and sex: 1976

Age	Number			Rate per 100,000 population in specified group		
	Both sexes	Male	Female	Both sexes	Male	Female
All ages	26,832	19,493	7,339	12.5	18.7	6.7
Under 1 year	...	...	...	...	...	...
1-4 years	...	...	...	...	...	...
5-14 years	163	126	37	0.4	0.7	0.2
15-24 years	4,747	3,786	961	11.7	18.5	4.8
25-34 years	5,064	3,716	1,348	15.9	23.6	8.4
35-44 years	3,759	2,557	1,202	16.3	22.8	10.2
45-54 years	4,541	2,990	1,551	19.2	26.2	12.7
55-64 years	4,005	2,826	1,179	20.0	29.8	11.1
65-74 years	2,772	2,094	678	19.5	34.0	8.4
75-84 years	1,406	1,096	310	20.8	42.7	7.4
85 years and over	371	299	72	18.9	47.5	5.4
Age not stated	4	3	1	...	...	...

Table 42. Death rates for Homicide by color and sex: Selected years, 1950-76

[Rates per 100,000 population in specified group]

Year	Total			White			All other		
	Both sexes	Male	Female	Both sexes	Male	Female	Both sexes	Male	Female
1976[1]	9.1	14.5	4.0	5.4	8.3	2.7	33.2	55.8	12.5
1975[1]	10.0	16.0	4.4	5.9	9.1	2.9	37.1	62.6	13.8
1974[1]	10.2	16.3	4.4	5.8	8.9	2.8	39.7	67.2	14.5
1973[1]	9.8	15.5	4.3	5.5	8.3	2.8	39.1	65.8	14.6
1972[1,2]	9.4	15.4	3.7	4.9	7.7	2.3	40.5	70.1	13.4
1971[1]	9.1	14.7	3.8	4.7	7.3	2.3	39.6	67.7	13.9
1970[1]	8.3	13.4	3.4	4.4	6.8	2.1	35.5	60.8	12.3
1969[a]	7.7	12.4	3.2	4.0	6.1	2.0	34.2	58.7	11.7
1968[a]	7.4	11.9	3.1	3.9	6.0	1.9	32.4	55.1	11.6
1967[a]	6.8	10.6	3.2	3.6	5.3	1.9	30.2	49.9	11.9
1966[a]	5.9	9.1	2.9	3.1	4.5	1.8	26.5	43.7	10.5
1965[a]	5.5	8.6	2.6	3.0	4.4	1.6	24.6	40.4	10.0
1960	4.7	7.1	2.4	2.5	3.6	1.4	21.9	34.5	9.9
1955	4.5	6.9	2.1	2.3	3.4	1.2	22.8	36.9	9.5
1950	5.3	8.1	2.4	2.6	3.9	1.4	28.0	45.5	11.2

[1] Excludes deaths of nonresidents of the United States.
[2] Based on a 50-percent sample of deaths.
[a] Revised.

Table 43. Death rates for Homicide by age and sex: 1976

Age	Number			Rate per 100,000 population in specified group		
	Both sexes	Male	Female	Both sexes	Male	Female
All ages	19,554	15,142	4,412	9.1	14.5	4.0
Under 1 year	170	88	82	5.6	5.7	5.6
1-4 years	306	154	152	2.5	2.4	2.5
5-14 years	392	240	152	1.1	1.3	0.8
15-24 years	5,038	3,907	1,131	12.4	19.1	5.6
25-34 years	5,266	4,264	1,002	16.5	27.0	6.2
35-44 years	3,288	2,666	622	14.3	23.8	5.3
45-54 years	2,371	1,882	489	10.0	16.5	4.0
55-64 years	1,466	1,140	326	7.3	12.0	3.1
65-74 years	759	549	210	5.3	8.9	2.6
75-84 years	362	180	182	5.3	7.0	4.3
85 years and over	97	41	56	4.9	6.5	4.2
Age not stated	39	31	8	...	...	...

☆ U. S. GOVERNMENT PRINTING OFFICE : 1978 621-546/251